AF698872

You Are What You Eat.....

Therefore let food be thy medicine

by

Cecilia Salvesen

Disclaimer: The author is a lifestyle health professional and holds diplomas in Complementary Medicine, Therapeutic Reflexology, Therapeutic Aromatherapy, and Anatomy, Physiology and Pathology. When consulting, she aims to identify the cause that may have created an imbalance, blockage or congestion within the body and advises accordingly. Advice given by her may differ from the theories and practice of the medical, or any other profession. She does not diagnose, prescribe or alter prescribed medication. Information contained in this book is based on her years of studies, experience and practice, and is entirely her own opinion. Readers are under no obligation to follow any advice given in this book, and should they have a serious or specific health problem, they are advised to seek counsel from any profession of their choice.

More information about the author is available at: www.ceciliasproducts.com

You Are What You Eat 3rd edition

ISBN 978-0-9842270-0-6

Published by: Lifestyle Institution LLC

Edited by: Shirley Ann Moon (South Africa)

Rosemary Howie (South Africa)

Sandra Ratto (USA grammar)

Edited and Indexed by: Cynthia Harvey-Williams (South Africa)

Formatting and Graphic Designs: Janene Salvesen (USA)

ACKNOWLEDGEMENTS

My sincere thanks to the following people:

My husband Errol Salvesen who has always loved and supported me in my work and career.

My son Conryd and **daughter Juanique** Salvesen who patiently allowed intrusion on family and private time on many occasions, thus enabling me to pay attention to clients and students at all hours.

Jessica Hart for continually and unselfishly being available to offer assistance.

Inge Dougans who introduced me to the concept of Acid/Alkaline foods.

Ruth Cockbain who made me aware of *Candida albicans*.

Joan Wilkinson who facilitated the healing of my body.

From the author:

As many people may read only certain chapters of the book applicable to their condition, I have reiterated important information and advice, if necessary and pertinent to that section.

When consulting with people and I mention the words “carbohydrates, proteins and fats” I am frequently asked to explain what those are. Consequently, I have taken the liberty to briefly describe these when mentioned.

Because this book is not meant to be read only, but is also intended to educated people who know very little about natural nutrition, I have recapped on many aspects, as repetition eventually instills understanding and knowledge.

Through these writings, I sincerely hope that many readers will realize the importance of our daily consumption, and that it truly leads to the final outcome of how and what we are.

Cecilia Salvesen

CONTENTS

CHAPTER 3

CHAPTER 4

CHAPTER 5

CHAPTER 6

CHAPTER 7

PREFACE

This book is dedicated to two women, one whom I don't know at all but only know of, and the other with whom I have, since our first encounter, become very friendly with over the past twenty-plus years.

The first woman is Ruth Cockbain who (at that time) lived in Pietermaritzburg, South Africa. Ruth is a member of our church and attended Pietermaritzburg ward and I, then living in Pinetown, South Africa, attend our local ward. Through the Youth Program, I had heard of Ruth (and vice versa), as her sons had attended youth activities and were friendly with my stepsons who attended the same activities.

The second woman is Inge Dougans who taught me the nutritional concept of Acid/Alkaline.

I had always considered myself a healthy person but soon after the birth of my daughter in December 1987, I started experiencing drastic changes in my body, mental alertness and emotional behavior. Soon I was losing weight at an alarming rate despite my constant hunger. I experienced tremors in my hands, nervousness, heat intolerance, palpitations, and alarmingly enough, slight exophthalmos (protrusion) of the right eye.

Early one morning in April 1988, I thought I was having a heart attack due to severe pains in the thoracic cavity and excessively rapid heart beat. Errol, my extremely caring husband, became alarmed at these very obvious changes and telephoned our doctor who ran a series of urgent blood tests. Due to the results I was referred to an endocrinologist who diagnosed me with Graves Disease which was at a life-threatening stage. Through the oral intake of Radio Active Iodine, the cells of my thyroid gland were destroyed, rendering it inactive. Left unmonitored for a few weeks, I plunged into hypothyroidism, which led to crucial Myxodema. My immune system was totally depleted and I was diagnosed, by the endocrinologist, with Myalgic Encephalomyelitis (M.E.). Almost comatose, I spent 6 days in hospital, fed intravenously, trying to recuperate, but to no avail.

I was discharged from hospital and was in a state where I could not walk up our front stairs. I had to pause three times to rest briefly while ascending the short flight of 16 steps. I could not lift my arms above my head to shampoo my hair (of which I had lost more than half due to Myxedema). I could not cross the room to answer the telephone, and I could not move my wrists to beat an egg and make scrambled egg for my (then) three-year-old son. I vividly recall making an attempt and dropping two eggs in succession before managing to break the third egg into a cup. I could not hold a pen and write my name. I felt as if I had been converted to slow motion as my actions and thoughts were decelerated. Apart from my son, my daughter was six months old and needed constant attention. She did not sleep at night (or during the day for that matter) and if I managed four hours broken sleep a night, I considered myself fortunate.

It was at this time that I received that life-saving phone call from Ruth Cockbain, who started her conversation as follows: "Cecilia, you don't know me, but I know of you and have heard that you have been very ill and have been diagnosed with M.E. My son was also diagnosed with M.E. and I would very much like to help you and offer advice. Have you heard of *Candida albicans* and are you aware that sufferers of M.E. have candidiasis due to their lowered immune system?"

I informed Ruth that I had never heard of candidiasis and spent the next half hour listening to her not only explain candidiasis, but also offering valuable advice on how to treat it through correct nutrition. After our conversation, I could not believe that an individual, whom I did not know but only knew of, had cared enough and taken the time to telephone me and offer such valuable knowledge and advice. I immediately took action and changed my diet accordingly.

My mother-in-law suggested I consult with the reflexologist who had successfully treated her and restored her health. Before my daughter was conceived, I'd had a reflexology treatment and was therefore not unfamiliar with the therapy. Joan Wilkinson is the wonderful reflexologist who used her therapeutic reflexology expertise and nursed me back to health. I received seven treatments in ten weeks and the reflexology treatments delivered by Joan Wilkinson, together with the anti-Candida diet as suggested by Ruth Cockbain, are directly responsible for the restoration of my health.

I was so impressed with what Joan had done for me that I decided (with encouragement from my husband) to pursue reflexology as a career. This is when I met Inge Dougans, who is the Principal and owner of the International School of Reflexology and Meridian Therapy. She is also the author of three books - some have been translated into eight languages. Inge is a world- renowned lecturer and gives lectures and workshops on reflexology throughout the UK, Europe and the USA. Although born in Denmark, Inge has lived in South Africa for many years.

I attended her school and learned the art of reflexology. She introduced to me the concept of Acid/Alkaline and the importance of natural foods. From there my interest grew and I proceeded with in-depth studies on nutrition, *Candida albicans,* the immune system and the effects of natural foods in fighting diseases.

This book is merely a synopsis, but the concept remains unchanged and unbelievably simple. We are what we eat, as we eat to sustain life (and not satisfy our taste buds). What we consume will ultimately become us - our hair, nails, skin, body secretions and structures. If we fuel our bodies with natural, nutrient rich foods, we can live a life that is dis-ease as well as disease free. If we fuel our bodies with refined, carcinogenic, chemical foods, we can expect to become either overweight or undernourished, often saddled with allergies and suffer from disease.

This book would not be justified without final acknowledgement to my husband Errol, my son Conryd and my daughter Juanique. They have fully supported me in my career and have spent many hours pursuing their own lives while leaving me to study, treat clients and educate therapists. Without their support, none of my achievements (however great or small) would have been possible. Errol has been my pillar of strength. He is my help-meet, my partner, colleague and friend. He is strong and wise yet he is the kindest and most gentle person I know. He has always been the perfect gentleman and I will remain eternally grateful to him for his devotion to our relationship and family unit.

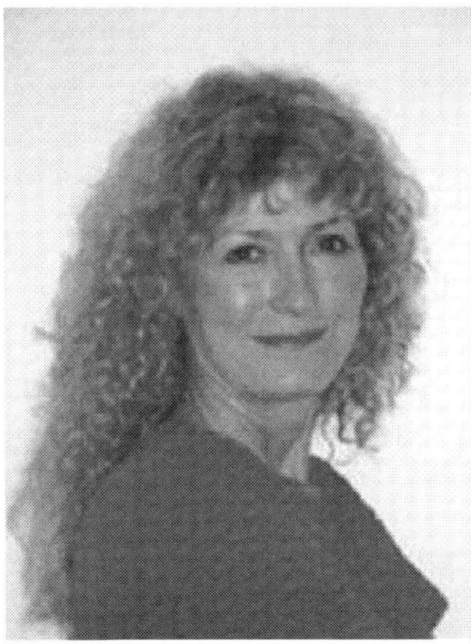

Cecilia Salvesen

FOREWORD

By: Jessica Hart (South Africa)

In 1988 Cecilia was diagnosed with M.E. ('Yuppie Flu'). Reflexology and nutrition brought her back into action again. The article which appeared in the April 1991 issue of 'YOU' magazine in South Africa described her condition. Today she is cured of M.E., lives a full and active life, and is able to guide other people experiencing ill health. It is Cecilia's policy not only to help the body heal itself but to educate people to help themselves through nutritional advice and healthy living habits.

Cecilia studied with the International School of Reflexology and Meridian Therapy, and qualified as a reflexologist and meridian therapist. Soon afterwards she qualified as an aromatherapist and went on to complete a course in advanced massage techniques. She has continued to increase her knowledge and has qualified as a Practitioner of Complementary Medicine.

In 1992 Cecilia started the Natural Health and Beauty College where she ran therapeutic aromatherapy courses, lectures on nutrition, *Candida albicans,* treating children's illnesses naturally and other subjects of interest until she immigrated to the USA in 2002 . She is often invited to give talks on the above subjects to various groups and organizations. In the same year Cecilia launched her range of beauty and health products under the name Natural Health and Beauty Products (www.ceciliasproducts.com) and these have proved extremely effective.

Since becoming a committee member of the South African Reflexology Society in 1990, Cecilia served as an executive committee member, vice chairperson and chairperson of this society. She was actively involved with the society in negotiating with government for the statutory registration of reflexology. Cecilia was the first president of the umbrella reflexology body The National Reflexology Association, through which the application was made. She is a founder member of the Aromatherapy Society of South Africa which was formed in 1997 and was an executive member, representing the society on the Integrated Health Liaison Committee (then a standing committee of the Chiropractors, Homeopaths and Allied Health Service Professions Council of South Africa) holding two portfolios as Liaison Committee representative and Education representative. Cecilia was awarded Honorary Membership for both the Aromatherapy Society of South Africa and the South African Reflexology Society in recognition of her valuable contributions to these societies. She was nominated and formally gazetted as a member of the Standards Generating Body (SGB) for the Integrated Health Professions, to assist in writing unit standards for therapeutic aromatherapy. She also serves on the Board of Directors of the International Council of Reflexologists as Vice President.

Another 'cap' Cecilia wore was that of Regional Director for the International School of Reflexology and Meridian Therapy for Kwa Zulu Natal where she instructed students in therapeutic reflexology, meridian therapy, anatomy, physiology and pathology, nutrition, business and listening skills.

Cecilia is the author of ***"Aromatherapy for Natural Health and Beauty"*** and ***"You Are What You Eat"*** and is an international speaker on nutrition, aromatherapy, reflexology and other health and lifestyle related subjects.

Article as it appeared in the

"YOU"

11 April 1991

magazine

BY LUCIA GOMES and MAGARET MORGAN

Mrs Cecilia Salvesen of Pinetown was told three years ago that she had Yuppie Flu. She swore that she wouldn't let the sickness get her down Her determination has paid off - today the mother of two is her old self again.

" I tried everything", she says.

" But I found that reflexology and the right diet were all that really worked for me."

At first the sickness sapped all her energy and zest for life, making her tired and listless, having to force herself to do just the essentials.

She had always enjoyed an energetic game of squash and was a keen golfer: now she had to rest three times on the flight of steps to her front door. It took her ages to cross the room to answer the telephone. Although she was in her 30s she felt and moved like an old woman.

"My chest felt tight, I was always cold and short of breath," she says. "It was as if my batteries had run down. The headaches were worse than anything I could ever have imagined. Every joint and muscle in my body ached; the backache was unbearable and my jaw muscles were so sore I couldn't chew. But the worst thing about ME is that no one can see the pain; to other people you look the picture of health."

Cecilia's doctor prescribed anti-inflammatory medication for the muscle pain, she received physiotherapy and was referred to an orthopaedic surgeon. She found it so difficult to concentrate that she even insisted on a brain scan. Eventually she was diagnosed as having M.E. Her doctor prescribed rest and stressed the importance of the correct diet. Cecilia contacted the M.E. awareness group in Durban to ask how she could best help herself and began to faithfully follow the recommended diet which forbids all sugar, colorants, preservatives and refined foods.

"I decided right from the start that I

wouldn't allow ME to control my life," she says. But it wasn't easy. Soon after her diagnosis she was admitted to hospital suffering from exhaustion and put on an intravenous drip for six days. The medication prescribed by her doctor made her feel a lot worse instead of better. She fainted as often as three times daily, had no appetite and rapidly lost weight.

Finally, at her wits' end she decided to follow her mother-in-law's advice and see a reflexologist.

"I would have tried anything. When I had the first treatment I was too sick to feel the difference, but I couldn't believe what happened after my second visit. For the first time in months I was so hungry I couldn't get home fast enough to make something to eat."

After seven treatments over 10 weeks her body had stopped aching, the headaches had disappeared and she felt far more energetic. Now Cecilia is so healthy that she's tackled something new - she has qualified as a reflexologist and is able to help others, including other ME sufferers.

Reflexology involves stimulating the body's reflex centers by massaging specific areas on the feet. "It encourages the elimination of toxins and stimulates the body to heal itself," Cecilia explains.

Today she still takes care not to overdo things - if she does, the pains flare up again, though far less severely than during her first two years as an ME sufferer. "Apart from not being able to play sport I lead a normal life,"

It needs to be noted that since this article was written in 1991, Cecilia has long since returned to a normal, active life, having graded in karate, playing golf (when possible), walking, scuba diving and other activities that interest her.

"COVER GIRL"

Since birth my daughter Juanique (pronounced French "Jeanique") has eaten as nature intended. She grew up eating natural foods.

She took fruit to school and did not eat refined food. Even at the age of six, when playing at friend's home, told their mothers what 'good' foods and 'bad' foods are. Fortunately for me, they had a sense of humor. When she was nine, she went to a birthday party. The mom told me that she noticed my daughter was not eating so she asked her why, and Juanique replied "I don't eat that kind of food". She asked what she would like and Juanique asked if she had salad. She quickly went to the refrigerator, got out lettuce, tomatoes, cucumber and onion and made a salad. She related how stunned she was that this little girl sat at the birthday table and got stuck into her salad, enjoying it as much as the other children enjoyed the junk food.

I was convinced by many people to remove the cover off my book with this edition and replace it with a photograph of Juanique as she truly depicts that we are what we eat. Everything she eats has become her hair, her skin, her nails and each other functional cell in her body. That same rule of nature applies to us all.

INTRODUCTION

THE CAUSE OF DISEASE

I have written this book in the hope of helping the reader to understand the causes that contribute to a lowered immune system, and in turn render the body in a state of dis-ease or disease. These writings are based on years of personal research, experience and practice, and are entirely my own opinion. Readers under no obligation to follow any advice given, but I sincerely hope that should they choose to do so, they will notice and appreciate the improvement in their health, and be motivated to continue on a new-found path of wellbeing, remembering that **you are what you eat**.

A lowered immune system (resulting from pH imbalances in the systems) is one of the main contributing factors to dis-ease and disease. Many different factors affect the immune system and cause it to lower or dysfunction, leading to the misunderstanding that these factors cause different diseases. There are many different types of disorder ranging from rheumatoid arthritis and irritable bowel syndrome, to cystitis and asthma. The pathology list is endless. The medical profession is able to group a set of symptoms and "attach a label" (diagnose), thereby making identification of that disorder possible. For example, rheumatoid arthritis could include painful, red, swollen and inflamed joints. Frequent, cloudy, painful urination is characteristic of cystitis. Thus, many people are under the impression that different diseases are caused by different factors. **Excluding hereditary disorders and injury, there is only one major contributor to diseases and dis-eases and that is the immune system in a state of imbalance.** If the immune system is strong, then diseases and dis-eases can be avoided or overcome.

Factors negatively affecting the immune system are inferior or polluted food, air and water. Chemicals are a major contributor to our food, air and water pollution and are readily absorbed by the skin, inhaled or ingested in various ways. Injuries, fatigue, emotional and physical stress (especially long term or continuous stress) are further culprits negatively influencing the immune system and leading to ill health.

Often I am asked why certain people may abuse their bodies for many years and not show any sign of deterioration. Yet others will treat their bodies with care and concern but fall ill at a relatively young age, or unexpectedly and severely experience illness - frequently with fatal consequences. The answer is fairly uncomplicated. Each person will suffer from a different dis-ease or disease, depending on their personal weaknesses, regardless of the cause. In other words, if twenty people were given, for a certain period of time, the same diet consisting of refined, chemical saturated food, their individual imbalances would manifest in different organs and systems of their body. Each person, according to their strengths and weaknesses, will be inflicted with illnesses compatible with their body, regardless of the fact that they consumed the same food. Three may complain of arthritis and two are rheumatoid while the third is osteoporotic; two more may suffer from constipation and another from acne, while the fourth is afflicted with irritable bowel syndrome. Why are we different and why do our nutritional habits affect us diversely? The answer lies in our personal strengths and weaknesses. Our immune system will respond according to how strong or weak it is.

There are 4 basic causes of weaknesses:

1) **Hereditary conditions *beyond* our control:**

a) **Congenital disorders** (beyond our control) are not necessarily genetic and develop from internal or external environmental conditions, the health of the expectant mother, or unknown conditions that affect the fetus (in-utero). Often a developing fetus is at risk of disorders or abnormalities such as congenital heart defects. Congenital disorders are not always genetic and are not always passed on from parent to child.

Congenital disorders may include anomalies such as minor abnormal body structures (third nipple, curved finger) or major body structures (deformities and birth defects).

Pectus excavatum (sunken chest) is a congenital defect that may establish at birth or at puberty. It may be purely congenital, or it may be a symptom of Marfan syndrome, which is a genetic connective tissue disorder.

b) Genetic disorders (beyond our control) caused by abnormal chromosomes, or single- and multiple- gene defects, are conditions or diseases that are transmitted from parents to children and are often passed from one generation to the next (and may even skip a few generations). There are thousands of diseases caused by a single gene disorder.

Genetic disorders include diseases such as sickle-cell anemia, muscular dystrophy and hemophilia, which is a bleeding disorder where there is a deficiency of one of the blood clotting factors necessary for coagulation of the blood. Color blindness, downs syndrome and dwarfism are further examples

2) **Hereditary conditions *within* our control** are, in many situations, an inherited weakened immune system caused by malnutrition that can be strengthened as the generations go forward *if* they continue with correct nutrition. Unfortunately, bad nutritional habits are often passed down through the generations, especially as daughters learn cooking (and baking) traditions from their mothers, or sons request recipes to be passed on to their wives. (These disorders are more "kitchen-etic" than "genetic!")

If two children inherit weak heart and lung functions from either or both parents, their lifestyles may further weaken or strengthen their condition. If one child grows up smoking and drinking, their heart and lung functions will not only remain impaired, but will deteriorate to (possibly) beyond repair. Life expectancy as well as quality of life could also be affected drastically. Astronomical medical bills are inevitable. This person's children stand to inherit the same weaknesses (or worse – depending on their partner's health and hereditary conditions). If the other child grows up living a healthy life, eating natural foods avoiding carcinogens from refined products, exercises and in general practices healthy living, their heart and lung functions will strengthen. They will have quality of life, low medical expenses and their children could be born with much stronger heart and lung functions (especially if they marry a partner who also follows a healthy lifestyle).

3) **Injury to the body** may be caused in various ways such as a motor vehicle accident, a fall, sports injury, self-inflicted injury, assault, burning accident or exposure to environmental pollutants. The area of injury is potentially weakened even after healing has taken place. When the body is subjected to trauma, malnutrition, food abuse or any other factor causing an alteration to the body's homeostasis, the area of injury (regardless of how long ago) is often the first area where disease or dis-ease will manifest. An example of this manifestation is arthritis or rheumatism developing from old bone or joint related injuries.

4) **Self abuse** resulting from insufficient quantities of nutritious foods or an excess of nutrient-depleted foods. Simply phrased - eating too much of the bad foods and too little of the good foods. The concept of health is misunderstood. It is important to comprehend the long and short term effects inflicted on the functioning of the body when refined and nutritionally depleted food, laced with chemicals, sugar and other carcinogenic agents are consumed. This is not done intentionally, but naivety and skillful marketing cause many to believe that the ingestion of food has no effect on our state of heal

Health is so simple that often we think it is impossible to obtain and retain it. For good nutrition we need proteins, carbohydrates, fats, vitamins, minerals and trace elements. All natural foods contain these. Food should be fun, smell and taste good and be a way of life (not a diet!). Too often we stress over what to prepare and "will our family eat it?" We turn to quick, easy, inexpensive meals due to time constraints and budget limitations - yet we spend a small fortune on junk food, medical bills and medication.

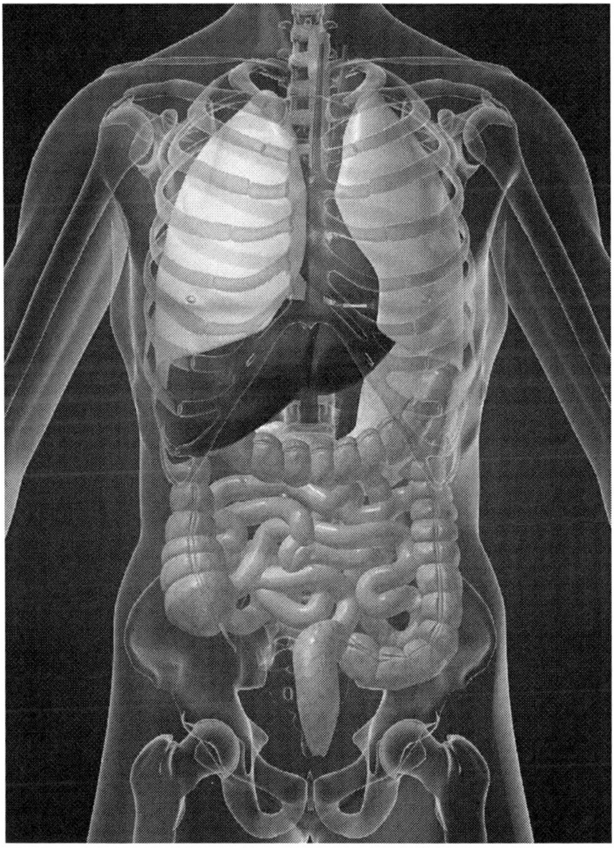

CHAPTER 1
NUTRIENTS

We classify food as either rich in nutrients or nutrient depleted. What are nutrients? There are six important nutrients necessary to sustain healthy life by ensuring cell growth, organ function, energy and homeostasis. These are: protein, carbohydrates, fats, vitamins, minerals and water. Without these, homeostasis will alter and dis-ease or disease will set in.

Protein, carbohydrates and fats are **macronutrients** as they provide energy. Vitamins and minerals are **micronutrients** and do not provide energy. All nutrients work together for one purpose: to sustain healthy life.

PROTEIN

Protein is converted into amino acids through the process of digestion, and is needed for building and repair of muscle, bone, skin, hair and nails as well as some hormone and enzyme production. Protein can be divided into **animal** and **plant**. Animal protein is found in dairy products (milk, yogurt, cheese, cream, butter), as well as meat, fish, poultry and eggs. Plant protein is found in nuts, seeds, pulses, grains and (unbeknown to most people) natural foods such as fruit and vegetables in varying degrees or amounts. Unfortunately, our major protein intake is animal and not plant derived, and therefore causes many dis-eases and diseases. Animal protein contains saturated fats that raise cholesterol levels, which is associated with heart disease. Excess animal protein causes many diseases, placing a strain on the liver, gall bladder and kidneys, and depleting minerals, while insufficient protein can cause the breakdown of muscle and tissue. Animal protein is not a clean burning fuel as most often their feed includes undesirable waste and byproducts. As we are what we eat, we too become what **they** eat. If we saw what many animals are fed, we would turn our head in disgust; yet we eat the animals' flesh which is made up of the byproduct feed they are given. There are twenty-two known amino acids; eight are essential (in their correct proportions), as they cannot be synthesized by the body and must be obtained from food.

ESSENTIAL AMINO ACIDS

Isoleucine, Leucine, Lysine, Methionine, Phenylalanine, Threonine, Tryptophan, Valine and Histidine.

SOURCES AND FUNCTIONS

Histidine: needed for growth, repair, and cell production. Essential for children and infants due to their growth spurts. Found in grains (wheat, rice, and rye), dairy, meat poultry and fish. (Histidine is an essential amino acid in infants but non-essential in adults).

Isoleucine: builds and repairs muscle tissue. Used in sport. Regulates blood sugar and formulates hemoglobin. Found in nuts, seeds, legumes, animal protein, eggs.

Leucine: works together with isoleucine and valine in protecting and healing muscle, bone and skin. Leucine has the ability to lower blood sugar levels. Found in brown rice, nuts, legumes, animal protein.

Lysine: needed for growth and bone development. Assists with calcium absorption. Found in yeast, animal protein, cheese, milk, egg, beans and potatoes.

Methionine: an antioxidant reduces histamine and breaks down fat. Found in seeds, lentils, beans, animal protein, fish, yogurt, garlic and onion.

Phenylalanine: used in the treatment of nervous disorders such as depression, lack of concentration and memory loss. Useful in pain control for conditions such as menstrual pains, arthritis, headaches and migraines. Found in animal protein, grains, legumes and dairy products.

Threonine: assists in producing anti-bodies that strengthens the immune system. Forms collagen and elastic fibers in the body. Found in animal protein and very little in grain.

Tryptophan: treats nervous disorders such as headaches, migraines, depression, mood swings, stress and insomnia. Found in legumes, grains, animal protein, and dairy products.

Valine: needed for repair and metabolism. Found in legumes, grains, animal protein, and dairy products.

NON-ESSENTIAL AMINO ACIDS

Non-essential amino acids are manufactured in the liver from other amino acids, and are thus not obtained through the diet. For this reason they are termed 'non-essential' even though they are extremely essential to the body. They are: Alanine, Arginine, Asparagine, Aspartic Acid, Cysteine, Cystine, Glutamic Acid, Glutamine, Glycine, Ornithine, Proline, Serine and Tyrosine.

FUNCTIONS

Alanine: assists with glucose metabolism.

Arginine: increases immune function activity and slows down developmental rate of tumors and other malignant diseases.

Asparagine: restores equilibrium to the central nervous system.

Aspartic Acid: assists with cell function, metabolism and increases endurance.

Cysteine: destroys harmful toxins. Responsible for strong appendages being skin, nails and hair.

Cystine: very similar to cysteine (described above). Has a rejuvenating effect on the body. Has the ability to clear blemishes and spots.

Glutamic Acid: valuable in treating disorders related to the muscular and nervous system such as epilepsy, learning difficulties, muscular dystrophy and many other conditions.

Glutamine: repairs and maintains muscle. Excellent for the nervous system. Supplements used in competitive sport as it builds muscle and protects the nervous system. Even though it is manufactured by the liver, it is available in raw green leafy vegetables.

Glycine: restores and repairs damaged tissue especially muscle and skin.

Ornithine: required for brain and liver function and to boost the immune system.

Proline: heals and repairs joints, tendons and muscle and skin.

Serine: builds up the immune system and aids with repair of the muscular system

Tyrosine: relieves stress conditions, mood swings, depression and other disorders related to the nervous system.

CARBOHYDRATES

Energy is essential to life, and carbohydrates are our main source of energy. In the digestive system carbohydrates are converted to glucose which is used and stored as energy (ATP- adenosine tri-phosphate) in the cells. The muscles, brain and nervous system in particular use a tremendous amount of the converted energy. Excess glucose is converted by the liver into glycogen and stored in the liver and muscles. Excess glycogen is then converted into fat and stored in adipose tissue, causing obesity and associated health disorders, as well as blood sugar diseases. Starches and sugars are the main source of carbohydrates, and are essential in moderation. Only when taken in excess or in a refined form do they pose a health threat.

Simple carbohydrates are high in calories and low in nutrients, as essential nutrients and fibers are removed during the refining process. Simple carbohydrates are found in fruit juices, refined sugars and flour, and processed products made with these ingredients such as bread, bread rolls, pasta, crackers, cookies, candies, chocolate, chips, soda pop, and other commercial foods. Refined carbohydrates provide instant but short spurts of energy resulting in lowered blood sugar.

Complex carbohydrates, found in fruit, vegetables, nuts, seeds, legumes and whole grains, ensure sustained energy and prevent hypoglycemia. Plant proteins are a good source of complex carbohydrates as the process of conversion is slower, providing a regular flow of sustained energy. Fruit is a healthy form of carbohydrates, as the fructose is rapidly absorbed into the blood stream producing instant energy. Fruit, depending on the amount of water, fiber and nutrients can be classified as either complex or simple - either are a natural good source of energy. Raw honey is hardly digested by us as it has been predigested by the bee and therefore enters the blood stream rapidly. Raw honey fights bacteria and is an excellent source of vitamins, minerals, protein and enzymes.

FATS

Fat is necessary for warmth, protection, building cell and nerve membranes. It also provides a form of energy and is needed to transport fat soluble vitamins (A, D, E, and K). Fat plays a major role in our body temperature homeostasis. It is required for the production and regulation of hydrophobic hormones (steroids) which are repelled by water. It is needed for the process of digestion, energy metabolism, memory storage and nerve impulses.

Several fats may promote health and are necessary in our diet, while others have a negative effect and excess can lead to heart disease and certain cancers. There are health-promoting fats and harmful fats. Four major fats dominate the foods we eat. These are: saturated fats, trans fats, monounsaturated fats and polyunsaturated fats. Regardless of which fat it is, each fat has 9 calories per 1 gram of fat. To better understand fats, I basically summarize them as *good* and *bad.*

<table>
<tr><th colspan="3">“GOOD” FATS</th></tr>
<tr><td colspan="3">UNSATURATED FATS</td></tr>
<tr><td colspan="3">Liquid at room temperature</td></tr>
<tr><td colspan="3">Lowers (LDL) (bad) cholesterol
Raises total and (HDL) (good) cholesterol</td></tr>
<tr><td colspan="3">Found in: Vegetables, plants and fish</td></tr>
<tr><td colspan="3">Divided into Polyunsaturated and Monosaturated fats.</td></tr>
<tr><td colspan="2">Polyunsaturated</td><td>Monosaturated</td></tr>
<tr><td colspan="2">Essential Fatty Acid (EFA). Must be obtain from the diet because it cannot be produced by the body</td><td>Non-Essential Fatty Acid because it can be produced by the body</td></tr>
<tr><td>EFA
Omega -3 oil
Alpha-Linoleic Acid</td><td>EFA
Omega -6 oil
Linoleic Acid</td><td>Non-Essential FA:
Omega -9 oil
Oleic Acid</td></tr>
</table>

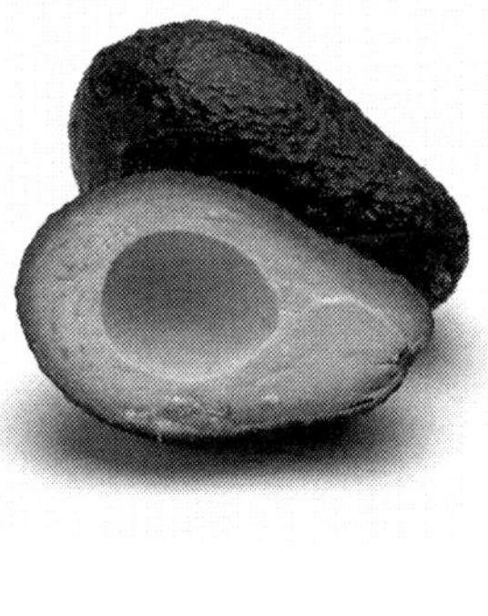

"BAD" FATS
SATURATED FATS
Solid at room temperature
Raises total and LDL (bad) cholesterol
Found in: animal, plant and processed foods

"BAD" FATS
TRANS FAT
Hydrogenated or partially hydrogenated oils.
Originally "good" unsaturated fats made "bad" by adding hydrogen gas to liquid fats to make them solid.
Not essential; Does not promote good health.
Hydrogenation prolongs shelf-life. Used in process foods: Microwave popcorn, French fires, potato chips, cookies, biscuits, pastries, pie crusts, donuts, pizzas, vegetable shortening, hard stick margarine

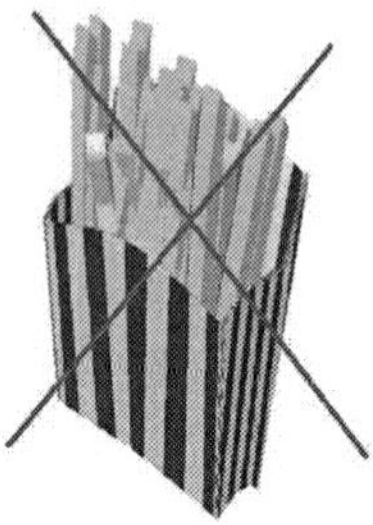

Herewith a further synopsis of fat we should, or should not eat:

UNSATURATED FATS

Unsaturated fats can be divided into polyunsaturated fats and monounsaturated fats.

POLYUNSATURATED FAT

Polyunsaturated fatty acids are liquid at room temperature and much more solid when cold (e.g. refrigerated). They have the possible ability to lower Low-density lipoprotein (LDL) (bad) cholesterol, and raise High-density lipoprotein (HDL) (good) cholesterol. Oils and food containing polyunsaturated fats, providing valuable Essential Fatty Acids (EFA) omega-3 and omega-6, which need to be obtained from the diet as the body cannot produce them. Oils and foods containing these fatty acids are:

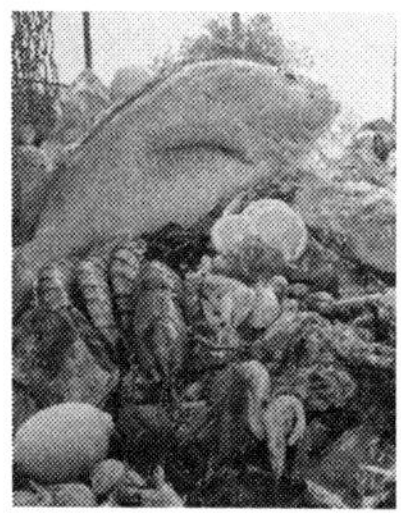

Omega 3: Cod, mackerel, herring, salmon pilchards, sardines, tuna, flaxseed, walnuts, dark green vegetables (kale, broccoli, spinach, lettuce).

Omega 6: Sunflower seed, safflower seed, evening primrose, borage, pumpkinseed, sesame seed, olives and olive oil, corn and corn oil, linseed, walnuts, almond and other nuts, hemp oil.

> Soy oil qualifies in this category but I don't support the use of soy oil, or soy products at all. I believe most soy available is Genetically Modified and that there is a link between soy phytoestrogens and breast cancer as these plant estrogens have the ability to disrupt the endocrine system.

MONOUNSATURATED FAT

Monounsaturated fatty acids are also liquids at room temperature but more solid in cold temperature. These fats also have the ability to lower Low-density lipoprotein (LDL) (bad) cholesterol, and may have the ability to raise High-density lipoprotein (HDL) (good) cholesterol. Monounsaturated fats contain Non- Essential Fatty Acids (non-essential because they can be produced by our bodies).

Oils and food containing monounsaturated fats are rich in omega-9 and found in:

- Fatty Acids (non-essential because they can be produced by our bodies).

Oils and food containing monounsaturated fats are rich in omega-9 and found in:

- Nuts (almond, hazel, walnut).
- Legumes (peanuts).
- Fruit (avocado, olive oil).
- Seeds (grapeseed, sesame, sunflower, safflower, chia, pumpkin).
- Grain (corn, wheatgerm).

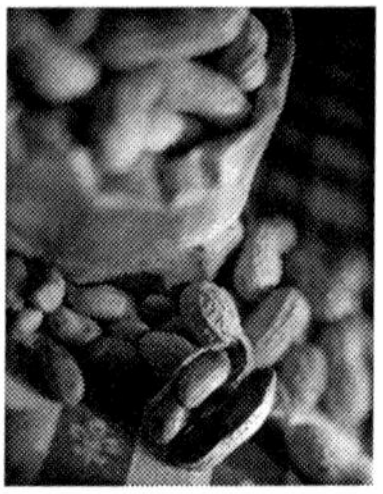

> Although canola oil qualifies in this category I don't support the use of canola oil at all. I believe it is Genetically Modified from rapeseed and the name is derived from "Canadian oil, low acid"

SATURATED FATS

- Saturated fats are hard or solid at room temperature and are not essential to health. These fats clog arteries and raise total and LDL (bad) cholesterol levels and should be avoided. Oils and food containing saturated fats are:
- Animal products: meat, cheese, eggs, milk, butter, cream.

- Processed foods: pastries, cookies, chips, deli meats.
- Plants: palm, palm kernel, coconut (hydrogenated), coconut (organic, virgin)

Organic, cold-pressed coconut oil has many health benefits but hydrogenated and partially hydrogenated coconut and palm oils are to be avoided. Hydrogenated oils are used extensively in the food industry as they do not go rancid quickly and they are cost effective. It is valuable to keep in mind that the inexpensive ingredients are not necessarily the healthiest ingredients. For this reason I have warned that money saved on inferior and chemical foods is often spent, ten times over, on medical bills at a later stage. Saturated fats increase cholesterol in the blood and contribute to heart disease.

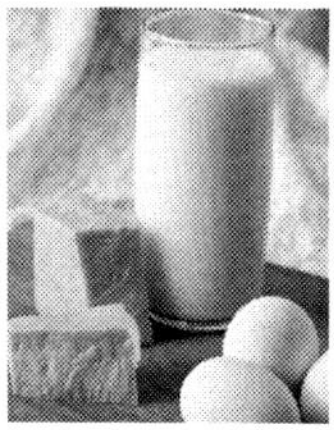

TRANS FATS

Trans fats, also know as trans fatty acids, are hydrogenated or partially hydrogenated oils which can be natural or synthetic. Very small amounts of natural trans fats can be found in animal products. Synthetic trans fats are formed when hydrogen gas is fused into heated unsaturated oils, using a metal catalyst (which allows oils to solidify) like nickel, aluminum, and cobalt to transform it from a liquid oil to a sold (hydrogenated) or semi solid (partially hydrogenated) fat.

Monounsaturated fat (non essential fatty acid) contains omega-9 fatty acid which is found in a variety of animal and vegetable foods. The process of hydrogenation delivers the saturated fatty acid - stearic acid which is used in making soap, candles, plastics, and cosmetics.

Commercial foods use trans fats because they are cost effective and prolong the shelf-life of processed foods. Trans fasts are not required by the body as they are (mostly) not natural and therefore not health promoting. Foods containing trans fats are: Microwave popcorn, French fires, potato chips, cookies, biscuits, pastries, pie crusts, donuts, pizzas, vegetable shortening, and hard margarine.

FIBER

Fiber is an indigestible food, which passes through the digestive system and is eliminated by the bowel. It contains no nutrients and its function is to absorb liquid and assist with the passing of stools which are made up of fiber and undigested food. Fiber ensures that the undigested food is moved through rapidly, thereby eliminating toxins and preventing bowel diseases such as diverticulitis, colon and rectal cancer. Hernias (hiatus, inguinal, umbilical, etc.) and gall stones may be prevented as well. A diet low in fiber can take as much as three days to pass through the system, whereas a high-fiber diet can take less than 24 hours. Processed foods are depleted in fiber and are thus a high contributor to colon related ailments. Natural foods such as vegetables, fruit, grains, beans, pulses (peas, lentils), nuts and seeds are the only good source of roughage. Gluten-containing products such as wheat, barley, rye and oats play a larger role in cleaning the intestines by more than just the fiber they provide. Gluten, as the name suggests, has a glue-like effect in the intestines where undigested foods stick to the paste, and are subsequently removed, preventing the fermentation and decomposition of undigested foods. Sweet corn is a richest form of fiber, together with yellow vegetables, which include all the squash and pumpkin family. Popcorn is a valuable snack as it not only provides fiber, but cleans the teeth. To ingest valuable fiber, it is important to not remove the peel from fruits and vegetables that do not require peeling. Washing these foods thoroughly is important.

Fiber is often divided into two groups i.e. soluble and insoluble fiber.

SOLUBLE FIBER comes from pectin in fruit (apples, oranges, strawberries, and gluten in grains (barley, oats). Whole grain cereals and beans provide gums which act as a fiber.

INSOLUBLE FIBER from bran, whole grains, seeds, leaves, stems, skins.

Water in the diet is necessary for fiber to fulfill its function.

WATER

Although water does not contain nutrients, it may contain minerals - depending on the source and lactation, which would cause it to vary tremendously. Surface water (streams, rivers, lakes) contains less dissolved minerals than ground water (wells, springs). Minerals the body requires, does not come from our water - it should come from our *natural* foods which absorbs minerals from the soil, which then becomes a usable source of minerals for our bodies.

Many people are confused about the internal use of distilled water as some say it is acceptable to consume and others say it is not. My personal preference is not to consume it, and these are my reason why I don't:

Distilled water is void of dissolved minerals and consequently has the ability to absorb minerals from the body, which may become a health hazard or even dangerous with prolonged use.

For this reason it is not recommended for drinking, especially prolonged use, and beverages made with distilled water should also possibly be avoided if given a healthier option. Because distilled water is an active absorber, it has the ability to absorb toxins from the body, which are eliminated through the urinary system, and is often used as a detoxifying agent. If we ate natural foods, we would not need to detoxify as these foods are rich in nutrients as well as antioxidants, which destroy free radicals. Due to it being an active absorber, distilled water (which may have a neutral pH), when exposed to air absorbs carbon dioxide, making it acidic. Approximately two thirds of the human body is made up of water, and it is essential to life as a person cannot survive more than a few days without replacing lost water. The body loses up to 3 liters of water per day (depending on body mass and activity) and this is mainly lost through exhalation, perspiration (±250 ml/1 cup), and urination which could account for more than 1 - 1.5 liters. Water is replaced with the natural foods we eat and the quality liquids we drink. **Quality liquids** are those found in natural whole foods (fruits and vegetables), purified or filtered water and herbal tea made with purified water using fresh or dried herbs.

An excessive intake of water can cause our systems to flush out valuable nutrients and place stress on our urinary system. Look at what nature gave us to drink as a natural source - water and water contained in our natural foods. For this reason, we should drink when we are thirsty and further obtain liquid from whole foods.

VITAMINS AND MINERALS

Vitamins and minerals, although only required in trace amounts, are essential for good health. They have no energy but are actively involved in the release of energy from the food we eat. A deficiency can cause many disorders, ranging from growth failure, scurvy, beriberi, dermatitis, anemia, muscle cramps and night blindness, to rickets.

Vitamins (**natural** or **synthetic)** can be obtained either from food or supplements. Vitamins in natural foods are natural, but vitamin supplements may be either natural or synthetic. Natural vitamins should be produced from high quality "live" raw ingredients that do not contain solvents, chemicals, sugar coatings, fillers and binders. Natural vitamins normally do not cause toxic reactions. Synthetic vitamins have many ingredients that are chemicals and coal tar derivatives.

What is the difference between organic and inorganic? Vitamins are **organic** as they contain carbon, while minerals are **inorganic** as they do not contain carbon. However, ferrous gluconate, ferrous peptonate and ferrous citrate are organic irons, but ferrous sulphate is an inorganic iron. The latter is often used to treat iron deficiency anemia but is also known to possibly destroy vitamin E

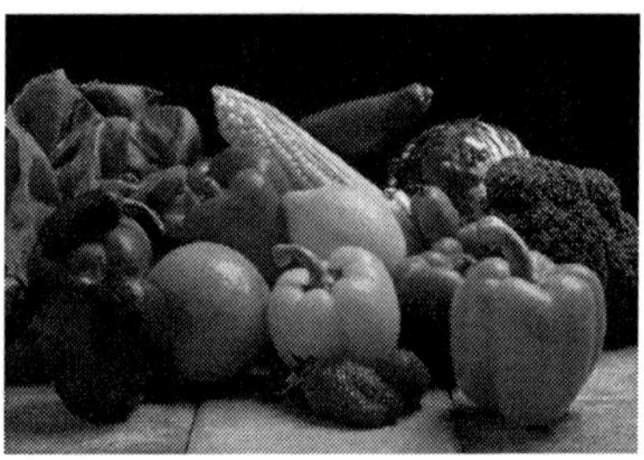

VITAMINS

Vitamins are organic compounds. There are thirteen major vitamins classified into two groups: **water-soluble** and **fat-soluble** vitamins.

WATER-SOLUBLE VITAMINS are the eight B complex vitamins (Thiamin (B1), Riboflavin (B2), Niacin (B3), Pantothenic Acid (B5), Pyridoxine (B6), Folic Acid, Biotin, Cobalamin (B12)), and vitamin C (ascorbic acid). These need to be taken daily as they are not stored in the body for any great length of time and the excess is excreted in urine.

FAT-SOLUBLE VITAMINS are A, D, E and K which are absorbed with other lipids (fat) and are stored in the liver and adipose tissue.

Vitamins are found in all natural foods and **no single natural food contains all the vitamins**. Hence it is necessary to eat a variety of foods, preferably those harvested within their season. The diet should provide vitamins as only certain vitamins can be produced by the body. Vitamin A can be synthesized by the liver from beta-carotene; vitamin D can be produced by the skin from the action of ultraviolet rays from the sun on a cholesterol compound within the skin; vitamin K, folic acid, biotin, thiamine, riboflavin and B12 are produced by the bacteria in the large intestine (colon). Although a component of natural foods, vitamins are separate from carbohydrates, fats, protein, minerals and water. They are present in most natural foods and are required by the body in very small amounts. Vitamins are essential for all the body functions and when there is a deficiency, they are known to cause a specific deficiency disease or syndrome.

Vitamins and minerals are both required as they assist each other in their functions. For example, vitamin C is required for iron absorption and activates folic acid; vitamin C is protected from oxidation by vitamin E; calcium requires magnesium to assist with absorption; and vitamin B12 requires the intrinsic factor from the stomach for the same purpose.

MINERALS

Minerals are inorganic nutrients and make up 4% of our body weight, while calcium and phosphorus, located mostly in bone and teeth, make up ± 75% of the mineral content. Minerals are ingested in the form of salts dissolved in food or water. Salts are required to maintain a fluid balance in the body and must be replaced by food and water (the latter to a lesser extent), as salts are naturally lost from the body through perspiration, urination and defecation. Salts are also lost, in vast amounts, from the body through diarrhea and immediate electrolyte replacement is crucial.

Minerals must be obtained from the foods eaten, as they cannot, like certain vitamins, be synthesized in the body. Minerals are normally classified into two groups as **macro** (major) needed in larger quantities, and **micro** (minor) needed in lesser or trace amounts.

MACRO MINERALS: Calcium, Phosphorus, Sodium, Chlorine, Potassium, Magnesium, Sulphur.

MICRO MINERALS: Iron, Copper, Molybdenum, Cobalt, Iodine, Selenium, Fluorine, Manganese, Zinc, Chromium.

OTHER MINERALS: Boron, Lithium, Nickel, Silicon, Tin, Vanadium, Arsenic.

MISCELLANEOUS MINERALS: Aluminum, Cadmium, Lead, Mercury.

ESSENTIAL VS. NON-ESSENTIAL: A mineral is not referred to as 'essential' unless a specific disease manifests which is corrected when the mineral is supplied.

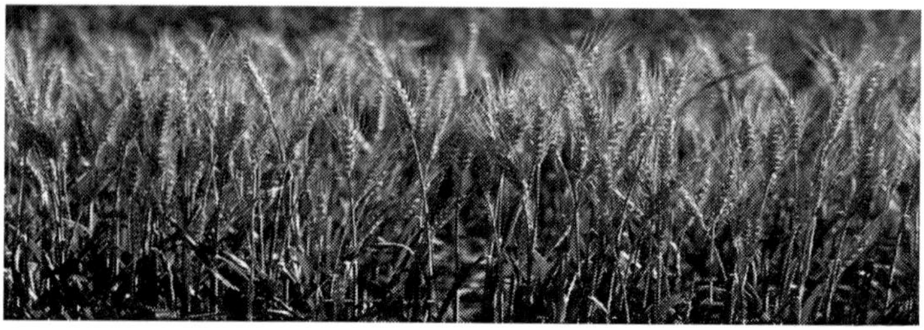

VITAMIN AND MINERAL CONTENT OF FOODS

FOODS RICH IN VITAMIN A		
Essential for good eyesight and eye disorders. Prevents night blindness. Important for clear and healthy skin. Promotes growth and is a cell regenerator. Necessary for strong nails, hair and teeth. Is an antioxidant and protects the body from cancer and other diseases including infections, especially of organs lined with mucous membranes. Used in the treatment of hyperthyroidism. Stores in the liver and can be toxic if used in excessively large amounts.		
apricots	egg yolk	parsley
asparagus	fish oil	peaches
beetroot	garlic	prunes
broccoli	kelp	Red peppers
butter	lemongrass	spinach
carrots	liver	spirulina
chives	milk	sweet potatoes
cod liver oil	mustard	turnip greens
cream	papayas	watercress
dandelion	paprika	yellow fruit
dark green vegetables	uncolored cheese	yellow vegetables

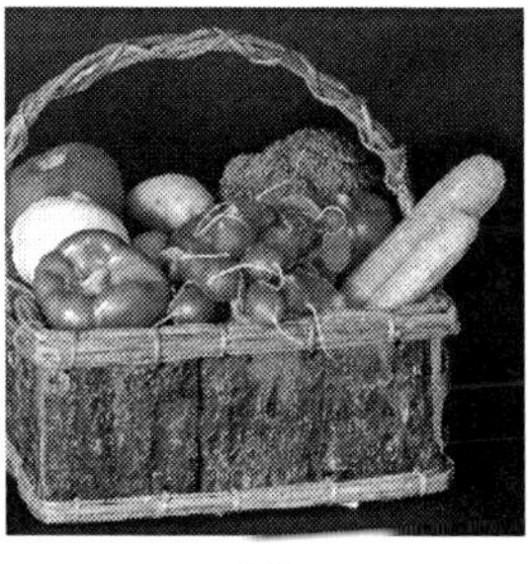

FOODS RICH IN VITAMIN B1 (THIAMINE)		
Important for growth. Stimulates digestion through the production of hydrochloric acid and increases carbohydrate metabolism. Aids nerve and brain functioning. Relieves motion sickness. Improves circulation. Also acts as an antioxidant, protecting the body against damage and disease.		
brewer's yeast	kelp	peanuts
broad beans	legumes	plums
broccoli	lima beans	raisins
brown rice	liver	red beans
brussels sprouts	meat	sesame seeds
cashews nuts	millet	soy beans
cereals	molasses	spirulina
chickpeas	mung beans	wheat germ
egg yolks	nuts	whole grains
fish	oat meal	yeast

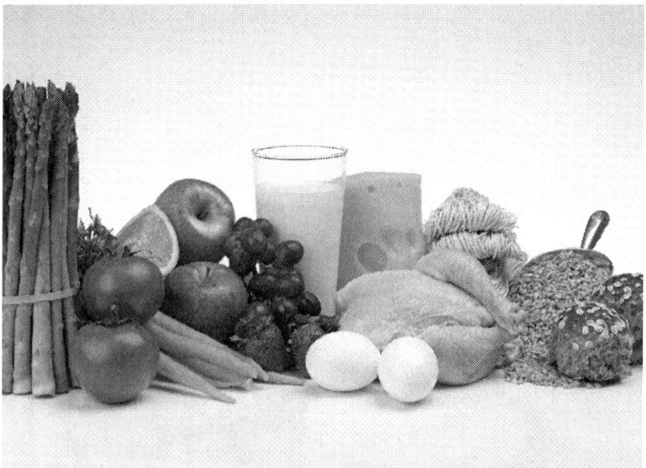

FOODS RICH IN VITAMIN B2 (RIBOFLAVIN)		
Essential for healthy skin, hair and nails. Plays a role in protein, fat and carbohydrate metabolism. Necessary for clear and healthy eyes preventing eye disorders. Is needed to strengthen the nervous system and aids with sleep.		
apricots	green vegetables	spinach
bran	liver	tomatoes
cheese	meat	wheat germ
chicken	milk	whole grains
eggs	poultry	yeast
Fish		

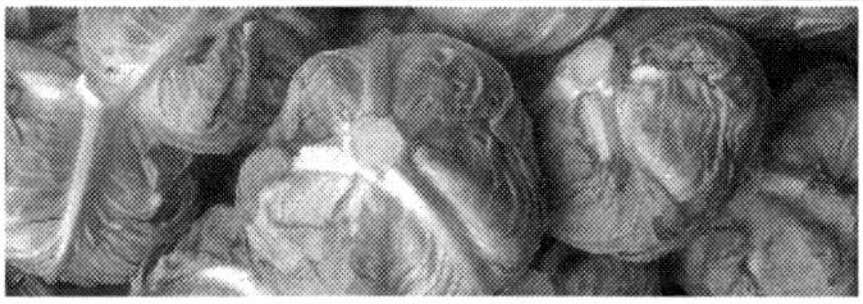

FOODS RICH IN VITAMIN B3 (NIACIN)		
Necessary for brain and nerve function. Aids in lowering cholesterol. Stimulates circulation. Promotes clear and healthy skin. Aids in metabolism and digestion.		
brewer's yeast	eggs	nuts
broccoli	fennel seed	parsley
carrots	fish	potatoes
Chamomile	lean meat	tomatoes
cheese	legumes	wheat germ
chicken	liver	whole cereals
Dates		

FOODS RICH IN VITAMIN B5 (PANTOTHENIC ACID)		
Major stress reliever and aids in synthesis of adrenaline. Calms the nervous system. Prevents anemia and formulates antibodies. Is an energy enhancer.		
beef	legumes	royal jelly
brewer's yeast	mushrooms	rye
eggs	nuts	vegetables
fish	organ meat	wheat

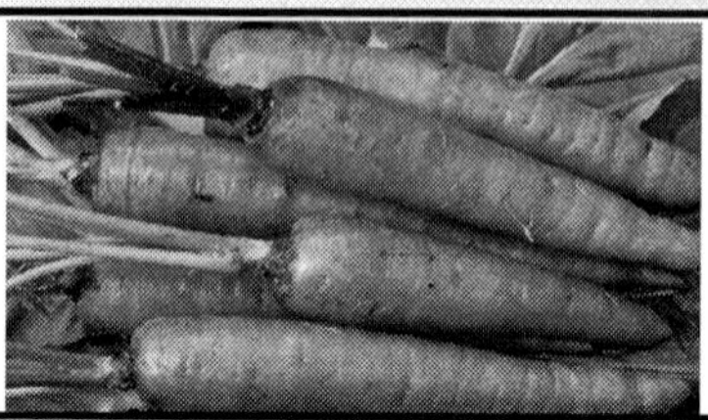

FOODS RICH IN VITAMIN B6 (PYRIDOXINE)		
Essential for assimilating protein in the body. Necessary for a healthy nervous system and brain functioning. Promotes healthy muscle and nerve tissue and is needed to prevent skin disorders such as acne and cracked lips. Reduces cramps and spasms		
avocado	egg yolk	peas
bananas	fish	seeds
beans	liver	soy beans
brewer's yeast	meat	soy flour
brown rice	milk	spinach
cabbage	molasses	wheat bran
carrots	nuts	wheat germ
chicken	oatmeal	

FOODS RICH IN VITAMIN B12 (COBALAMIN)		
Necessary for red blood cell production. Aids digestion. Helps memory, learning and brain fatigue. Improves balance. Needed to maintain a strong nervous system.		
brewer's yeast	kelp	milk
cheese	kidneys	oily fish
dairy products	liver	soy beans
eggs	meat	wakame (seaweed)

FOODS RICH IN VITAMIN B13 (OROTIC ACID)		
Necessary for good circulation. Supplies oxygen to the heart and blood cells thereby keeping it healthy. Detoxifies the liver and other organs. Delays aging.		
apricot kernels	liquid whey	sunflower seeds
brewer's yeast	root vegetables	whole grains
brown rice		

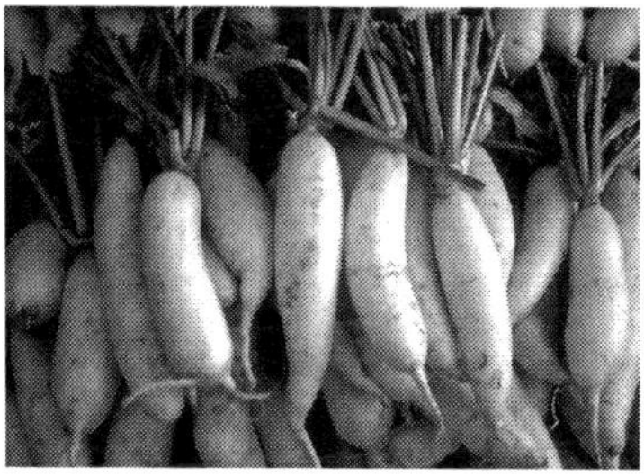

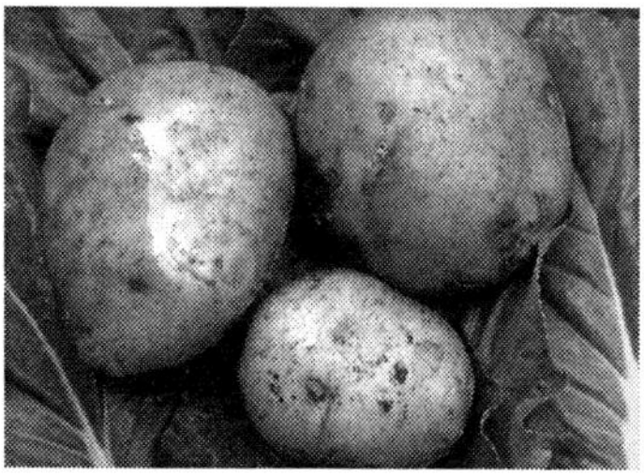

FOODS RICH IN FOLIC ACID (FOLACIN)		
Prevents anemia. Important for formation of red and white blood cells. Invaluable for a healthy pregnancy as it prevents birth defects such as spina bifida. Assists with lactation. Is an analgesic. Needed for healthy hair and skin and retards graying of hair. Assists cell activity, division and replacement. Treats depression and anxiety and is a food source for the nervous system. Eases insomnia. Needed for normal brain functioning especially for the fetus when pregnant. Promotes sound digestion and prevents digestive disturbances such as parasites.		
animal protein	dates	mushrooms
apricots	fish	nuts
avocados	grains	other whole grains
barley	green vegetables	potatoes
bran	kidneys	pumpkin
brewer's yeast	green leaf vegetables	root vegetables
brown rice	legumes	rye
Carrots	lentils	split peas
citrus fruits	liver	wheat germs
dairy products	melon fruits	

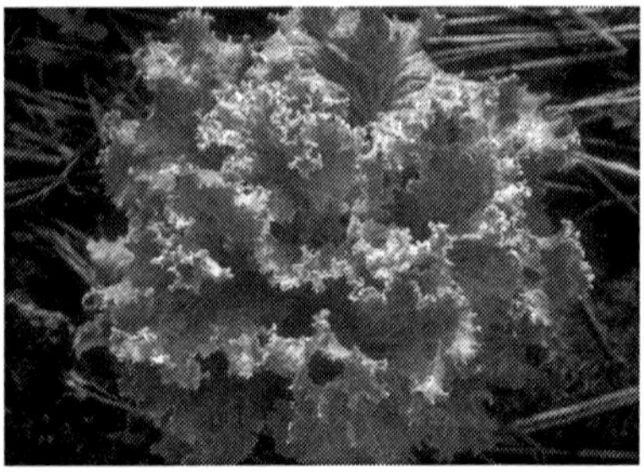

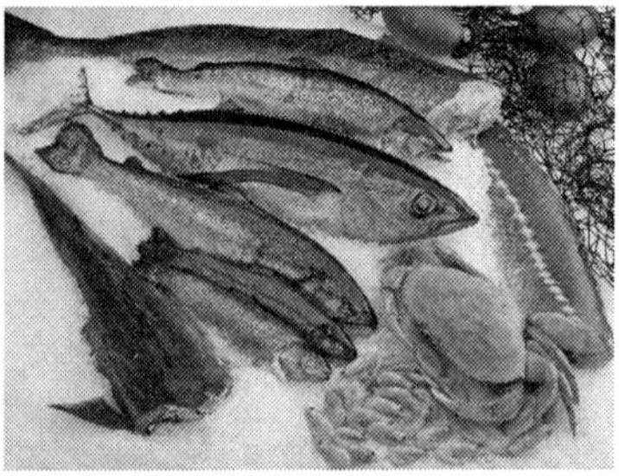

FOODS RICH IN VITAMIN C (ASCORBIC ACID)		
Essential for production of healthy connective tissue, good bone structure. Prevention of infection and fighter of respiratory and other infections. Prevents viral infections as well. Assists iron absorption. Prevents vitamin C deficiency disorders such as scurvy. Heals wounds, cuts and abrasions. Heals burns. Lowers cholesterol and high blood pressure (hypertension). Helpful in the treatment and prevention of thrombosis. Valuable antioxidant especially combined with vitamins E and A.		
all berries	green vegetables	peas
all citrus fruits	kelp	pineapples
blackcurrants	lemons	potatoes
broccoli	mangoes	radish
brussels sprouts	mint	rosehip
cherries	onions	sprouting seeds
chili peppers	oranges	strawberries
fresh fruit	papayas	tomatoes
grapefruit	parsley	watercress
green peppers		

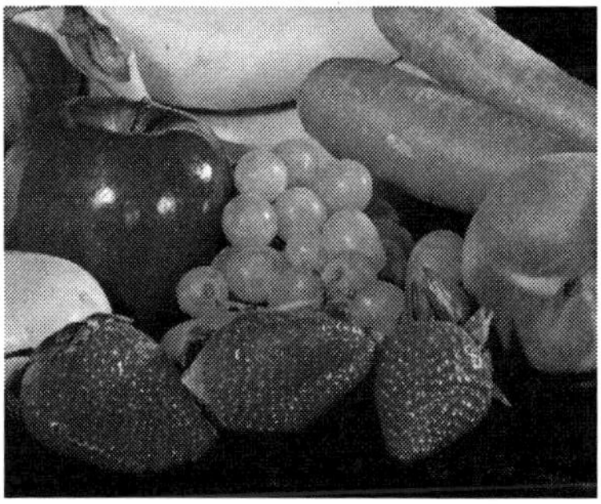

FOODS RICH IN VITAMIN D (SUNSHINE VITAMIN)		
Vital for the formation of healthy bones and teeth. Assists with insomnia. Aids good vision. Needed for calcium and phosphorous absorption. Strengthens muscles. Aids blood clotting. Prevents osteomalacia and rickets. Called the sunshine vitamin as the body synthesizes large amounts of vitamin D through sunshine.		
alfalfa	cod liver oil	milk
all fish products	eggs	oatmeal
butters alfalfa	fish	parsley
cheese	liver	sweet potatoes

FOODS RICH IN VITAMIN E (TOCOPHEROL)		
Excellent antioxidant, making it an anti-aging vitamin. Necessary for healthy blood vessels, nerves and muscles. Aids healing of damaged skin and tissue. Needed for healthy hair. A treatment for cuts, wounds and burns - also reduces scarring. Prevents eye disorders such as cataracts. Prevents anemia and miscarriages. Reduces fatigue.		
alfalfa	heart	oatmeal
avocados	kelp	rosehip
brown rice	kidney	seeds
butter	liver	sweet potatoes
cold-pressed oils	milk	wheat germ
dandelion	molasses	whole cereal
eggs	nuts	whole grains
flaxseed	green leaf vegetables	

FOODS RICH IN VITAMIN K (MENADIONE)		
Blood clotting factor and necessary for proper blood formation. Necessary in the prevention of internal hemorrhages such as ulcers, hemorrhoids and fissures. Valuable for bone formation. Is a tonic for the liver. Prevents infection. Also produced by friendly bacteria in the large intestine. Prevents bruising.		
alfalfa	fruit	oatmeal
broccoli	honey	rye
brussels sprouts	kelp	soy beans
cabbages	liver	tomatoes
cauliflower	molasses	Wheat germ
egg yolk	green leaf vegetables	
fish liver		

FOODS RICH IN VITAMIN P (BIOFLAVONOIDS, RUTIN)		
Fights infection. Maintains healthy blood capillaries and strengthens blood vessels. Reduces and prevents bruising. Acts as an analgesic, especially muscular. Assists the absorption and effectiveness of vitamin C. Reduces bleeding gums and other mouth disorders such as ulcers and herpes. Fights bacterial infections.		
alfalfa	dates	raisins
apricots	grapes	rosehip
blackcurrants	prunes	walnuts
buckwheat	green & red peppers	
cherries		

FOODS RICH IN CALCIUM		
Necessary for healthy bones, nails and teeth. Tonic for the nervous system. Prevents palpitations and regulates heartbeat. Helps with insomnia. Has analgesic effect. Prevents gum infections. Lowers cholesterol thereby preventing associated disorders. Prevents bone diseases such as osteoporosis and rheumatoid arthritis. Food source for the muscular system and alleviates muscle cramp and spasm. Eliminates fatigue. Needs to be taken with magnesium, which aids the absorption of calcium.		
almonds	eggs	sardines
asparagus	figs	sesame seeds
brazil nuts	goat's milk	soy beans
brewer's yeast	kelp	tofu
broad beans	milk	tuna fish
broccoli	molasses	watercresses
buttermilk	mung beans	wheat bran
cabbage	olives	whey
cheese	parsley	yogurt
chickpeas	prunes	
dandelion leaves	green leaf vegetables	

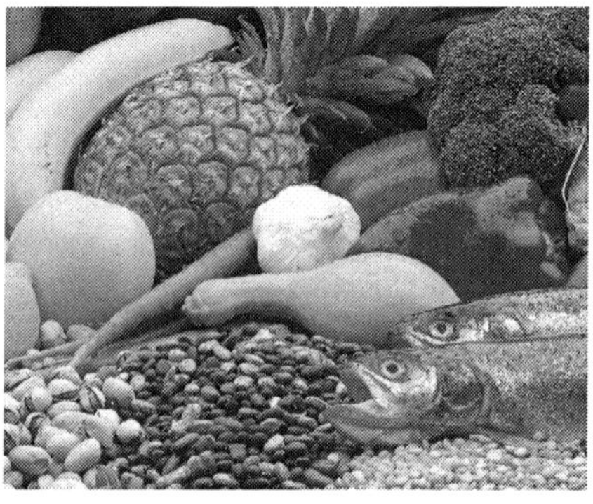

FOODS RICH IN MAGNESIUM		
Needed for the proper absorption and utilization of potassium, calcium, vitamin C and B6. Together with calcium it reduces the risk of osteoporosis, cardiovascular diseases. It plays a role in the prevention of certain cancers. Aids in the growth and repair of cells. Needed for muscle and nerve function. Needed in pregnancy and nursing of infants. Alleviates depression. Tonic for the heart and circulatory system. Aids digestion thereby eliminating indigestion.		
almonds	corn	nuts
apples	diary products	peaches
apricots	dates	peas
avocados	figs	seeds
bananas	fish	soy beans
beans	garlic	tofu
brazil nuts	kelp	wheat bran
brewer's yeast	green leaf vegetables	wheat germ
brown rice	lima beans	cashew nuts
meat	citrus fruits	molasses

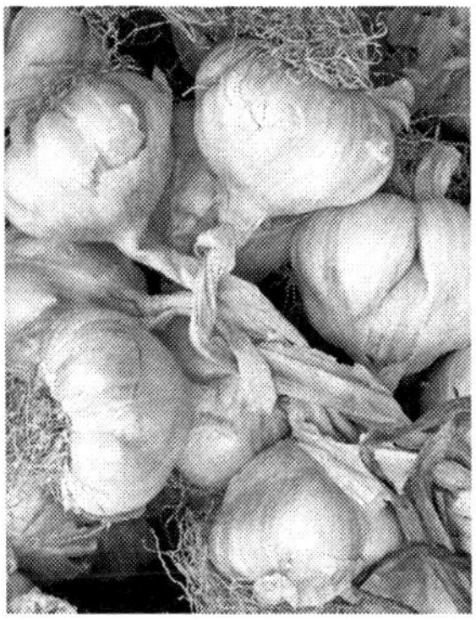

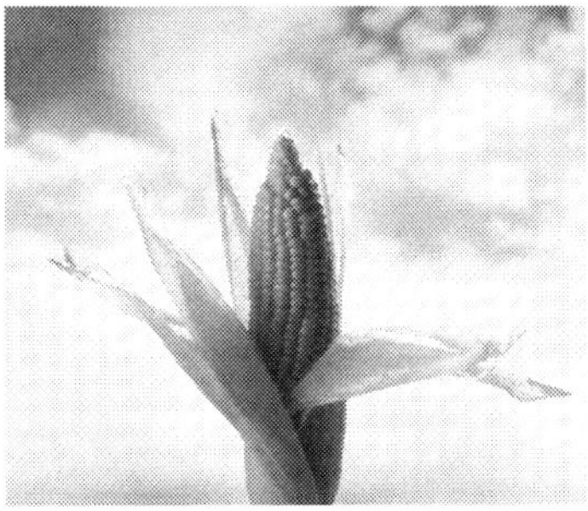

FOODS RICH IN POTASSIUM		
Anti-oxidant and detoxifies the body. Nerve and heart tonic. Prevents low blood pressure. Potassium and sodium levels are regulated by aldosterone hormone secreted by the adrenal cortex, causing the body to retain sodium and secrete potassium. Thus it plays a roll in controlling blood pressure and fluid balance. Relieves allergies. Alleviates cramps. Clears skin conditions.		
apricots	dried fruits	nuts
avocados	figs	potatoes
bananas	fish	poultry
brewer's yeast	fruit	raisins
brown rice	garlic	sunflower seeds
citrus fruits	legumes	vegetables
dairy products	meat	watercress
dates	molasses	whole grains

FOODS RICH IN IRON		
Essential for the correct functioning of oxygen in the body and for a healthy pregnancy.		
almonds	kelp	red peppers
beef	kidneys	soy beans
cashew nuts	lima beans	squash
dandelion leaves	liver	sun-dried apricots
egg yolk	molasses	sunflower seeds
eggs	pistachio nuts	wheat bran
green vegetables	pumpkin	

FOODS RICH IN SELENIUM		
Anti-oxidant - protects against certain carcinogens. Prevents prostate disorders. Works well with vitamin E in prevention of disease. Reduces the risk of hardening of the arteries. Slows down aging. Excellent for the skin and related conditions such as acne. Preserves the elasticity of tissue. Relieves menopausal symptoms (hot flushes). Selenium levels in food depend largely on the selenium content in the soil of countries where plants grow.		
alfalfa	ginseng	parsley
brewer's yeast	kelp	poultry
broccoli	lemongrass	vegetables
brown rice	liver	wheat germ
dairy products	molasses	whole grains
fish	nuts	yeast
garlic	onions	

FOODS RICH IN SODIUM		
Excessive intake of sodium will result in potassium depletion, edema and high blood pressure. Regulates water and blood pH balance. Necessary to replace when lost through heat and perspiration. Aids nerve and muscle function. Regulates low blood pressure.		
animal protein	herbs	seeds
beef	legumes	shellfish
carrots	nuts	soy beans
dairy protein	organ meat	tofu
fruit	salt	vegetables

FOODS RICH IN ZINC		
Zinc is required for the correct utilization of vitamin A in the body and assists with insulin formation and activity. Reduces infertility and prostate imbalances. Necessary for development of reproductive organs and the skeletal and nervous system of a fetus. Regulates blood pH balance. Zinc is depleted with extreme sweating. Heals wounds, cuts and burns. Prevents white spots found on nails. Restores sense of smell and taste. Lowers cholesterol.		
alfalfa	kidneys	rye
animal protein	legumes	sage
brewer's yeast	lima beans	seafood
brown rice	liver	soy beans
cheese	mushrooms	sunflower seeds
crab	parsley	walnuts
egg	pecan nuts	wheat bran
fish	poultry	wheat germ
kelp	pumpkin seeds	whole grains

Please note soy beans, soy flour and related products refer to organically grown soy beans and not genetically engineered varieties. The same applies to wheat grain, wheat germ and wheat bran.

Although I have listed soy and wheat for educational reasons, I do not promote the consumption of soy bean and soy bean products and caution people strongly on excessive intakes of wheat and wheat products. Reasons are discussed under 'FOODS TO AVOID' in Chapter 2.

CELL (TISSUE) SALTS

The human body is described as being **multi-cellular** as it is made up of millions of cells, and each cell is a living unit. Cells are made from the food we eat, which can be classified as **organic** and **inorganic**. **Organic materials** are protein, carbohydrates and fat. **Inorganic materials** are water and some minerals otherwise referred to as 'cell salts'. Cells differ in composition according to the type of tissue they form, e.g., nervous tissue is different from muscular tissue or cells forming bone. Skin is also different from any of the other cells mentioned. Mineral salts are cell builders. Materials for body growth and repair are supplied by the foods we eat (or should eat). Under normal circumstances we should obtain the necessary mineral salts from the foods we eat, but if our foods are dead or depleted, our bodies will eventually become depleted of the mineral salts lacking in our food. A homeopath, Dr. Wilhelm Schuessler, claimed that abnormalities and disease often resulted from a deficiency (or occasionally an excess) of one or more of these salts. He recognized symptoms as the body's distress signals and warnings that important constituents of the body were depleted or deficient. By providing for the need, the symptoms disappeared and the body normalized. He believed that by taking the correct salt, the body would receive the message and would then absorb the salts naturally. He also recognized that occasional excess could cause the same symptoms, and where there was an excess existing, when given to the body in smaller potencies, the body would still normalize the condition. Because excess can cause the same symptoms as deficiency, I recommend that cell (also known as tissue) salts only be taken sublingually until initial symptoms dissipate and then be discontinued. I believe that excessive use will negatively provide the body with "a crutch to lean on".

There are twelve main cell salts with specific effects on the body. Cell salts are completely harmless, and are safe and effective when treating children or people currently on medication, as they will not interfere with any form of drug. As with water-soluble vitamins, the body will discard what it does not need. The most effective way of absorbing the salts is through the buccal cavity. The mouth is lined with the buccal membrane and the absorption of substances through this membrane is rapid. Underneath the buccal membrane are tiny capillaries through which the substances are absorbed. The area underneath the tongue is dense with these capillaries; hence it is recommended that tissue salts be dissolved under the tongue.

It is important not to touch the tissue salts and for that reason they should be poured into the lid (cap), and from the lid popped into the mouth, underneath the tongue.

It is further important to mention that **Silica, the #12 tissue salt, should not be taken if there are foreign objects in the body such as steel plates, pins or any other solid transplanted matter**. Silica is an eradicator and will eliminate all foreign matter from the body. Thus it is excellent for detoxifying the body of metal, asbestos, chemicals and any other form of toxic substances.

SUMMARY OF FUNCTIONS AND SYMPTOMS RELATED TO THE 12 CELL SALTS

1. CELL SALTS	**CALC FLUOR**
COMMON NAME	CALCIUM FLUORIDE
LATIN NAME	CALCAREA FLUORICA
Function: **Elastic tissue** builder for blood vessels, skin, muscles. Strengthens tissue, restores and maintains tissue elasticity.	
Symptoms: Low muscle tone, loss of tissue elasticity (including blood vessels), stretch marks, muscular weakness, poor circulation, dental decay, loose teeth, cracks and fissures in the skin (including cracked heels, rectal fissures, and hemorrhoids), varicose veins.	

2. CELL SALTS	CALC PHOS
COMMON NAME	CALCIUM PHOSPHATE
LATIN NAME	CALCAREA PHOSPHORICA

Function: A constituent of **bones** and **teeth**. Aids formation of blood cells. Improves the health of bones. Expedites the healing of injured bones and tendons. Prevents hemorrhaging. Aids indigestion

Symptoms: Weak or diseased bones, ill-nourished states, simple anemia, poor circulation, numbness, chilblains, lowered vitality, lack of endurance, fatigue, teeth disorders, menstrual cramps.

3. CELL SALTS	CALC. SULPH.
COMMON NAME	CALCIUM SULPHATE
LATIN NAME	CALCAREA SULPHURICUM

Function: **Blood purifier**; constituent of blood and cleanser (detoxifies the liver).

Symptoms: Has a cleansing action and is beneficial for skin ailments: abscesses, boils (including gum boils), eczema, psoriasis, pimples, mouth ulcers, acne, and wounds that are slow to heal. Works well with Kali Mur (for inflammatory conditions) and Nat Sulph (in cleansing the liver).

4. CELL SALTS	FERR PHOS
COMMON NAME	FERRUM PHOSPHATE
LATIN NAME	FERRUM PHOSPHORICUM

Function: **Oxygen carrier** - oxygenates blood. Anti-inflammatory for all conditions of inflammation (sinusitis, cystitis, bronchitis, colitis, laryngitis, mastitis, arthritis, rheumatism, bursitis, gout).

Symptoms: Inflammation. Respiratory conditions and congestion (coughs, colds, influenza, bronchitis, catarrh, tonsillitis, sore throats, wheezing).Throbbing headaches, feverishness, rapid pulse, bleeding. To arrest bleeding, apply topically (in powder form).

5. CELL SALTS	KALI MUR
COMMON NAME	POTASSIUM CHLORIDE
LATIN NAME	KALIUM MURIATICUM

Function: **Blood conditioner.** Stimulates cell activity and helps with inflammation. Acts as a decongestant and aids respiratory disorders.

Symptoms: Congested conditions, thick whitish discharges, respiratory ailments, wheezing, coughs and colds, thickened blood, menstrual irregularities, white tongues. The children's remedy for coughs and nasal congestion.

6. CELL SALT	**KALI PHOS**
COMMON NAME	POTASSIUM PHOS
LATIN NAME	PHATEKALIUM PHOSPHORICUM

Function: **Nerve nutrient.** Aids the nervous system, tones muscles and prevents nerve degeneration. Use with Mag Phos.

Symptoms: Nervous exhaustion, brain-fog, depression, fretfulness, nervous headaches, bed-wetting, fatigue, tension, memory loss, lack of concentration and co-ordination, attention deficit, irritability, tantrums, insomnia, and other nerve related complaints. Aid in the healing of nerve and brain damage. Has proven beneficial to sufferers of Alzheimer, Parkinson's, stroke victims, cerebral palsy, Bell's palsy, shingles, neuralgia, trigeminal neuralgia, neuropathy and related conditions.

7. CELL SALTS	**KALI SULPH**
COMMON NAME	POTASSIUM SULPHATE
LATIN NAME	KALIUM SULPHURICUM

Function: Oxygenates cells and maintains healthy **skin, hair, scalp** and **nails.** A skin and mucous membrane conditioner.

Symptoms: Skin ailments and disorders of the scalp, hair and nails. Strengthens brittle nails and thinning hair. Aids mucous membranes; is an expectorant for catarrh; clears sticky discharges, and lowers the rise of body temperature in evening. For brittle nails and thinning hair, alternate with Silica No.12.

8. CELL SALTS	MAG PHOS
COMMON NAME	MAGNESIUM PHOSPHATE
LATIN NAME	MAGNESIA PHOSPHORICA

Function: **Nerve stabilizer**. Enables cells to eliminate waste. Relaxant and anti-spasmodic. Use with Kali Phos

Symptoms: Spasm, darting pains, "growing" pains, cramps, sciatica, menstrual pain, palpitations, nerve related toothache, flatulence, neuralgia, menstruation pains, renal colic, spastic colon, hiccups. Will act more rapidly if taken with a little (slightly) hot water

9. CELL SALTS	NAT MUR
COMMON NAME	SODIUM CHLORIDE
LATIN NAME	NATRUM MURIATICUM

Function: **Water distributor.** Regulates distribution of water from areas of excess (e.g. edema) to areas of "dryness" (e.g. eyes, mouth, vagina). Also regulates the distribution of red blood cells. Use with Nat Sulph.

Symptoms: Dryness or excessive moisture in any part of the body, running nose/colds, post nasal drip, loss of smell and taste, thin watery blood. Constipation (due to lack of fluids)

10. CELL SALTS	**NAT PHOS**
COMMON NAME	SODIUM PHOSPHATE
LATIN NAME	NATRUM PHOSPHORICUM
Function: **Acid neutralizer.** Neutralizes lactic and uric acid, prevents cholesterol crystals forming.	
Symptoms: Acidity, 'tummy' upsets, heartburn, malassimilation, indigestion, rheumatism (swollen and stiff joints), gout. Acidic blood conditions (pH)	

11. CELL SALTS	**NAT SULPH**
COMMON NAME	SODIUM SULPHATE
LATIN NAME	NATRUM SULPHURICUM
Function: **Water eliminator.** Eliminates excess water. Use with Nat Mur. Stimulates bile, balances level of water in body; is an excess water and acid eliminator.	
Symptoms: Biliousness, liver and gallbladder upsets (hepatitis, jaundice, cirrhosis), influenza, water retention, toxic states, bitter taste in the mouth. The 'liver salt'.	

12. CELL SALTS	**SILICA**
COMMON NAME	SILICONE DIOXIDE
LATIN NAME	SILICA
Function: **Cleanser and eradicator.** Firms tissue, eliminates pus, detoxifies.	
Symptoms: Pus formation, boils, abscesses, styes, scalp disorders, pimples and spots. For brittle or cracked nails, alternate with Kali Sulph.	
Caution: **Do not use if implants or foreign matter is purposely placed inside the body. Silica is an eradicator and foreign matter (and implants) may be expelled.**	

CHAPTER 2
GUIDELINES TO HEALTHY EATING

Eat as nature intended and keep food whole. Natural foods that have not been processed contain all the original nutrients and are free of preservatives, additives and other chemicals. Where possible, eat organically grown fruits and vegetables, as they should be free of chemicals. Many natural foods are sprayed so do wash them. Poultry and eggs should be from cage free chickens and meat from grass-fed animals not injected with growth hormones or steroids. Although general guidelines and advice is expanded upon in more detail, not all situations can be covered fully.

GENERAL ADVICE

APPLE CIDER VINEGAR is rich in potassium. A recommended drink to have morning and evening, is 2 teaspoons pure, organic apple cider vinegar and 2 teaspoons raw honey in a glass of water (optional: *warm* water - not hot or boiling. Temperature should not exceed body temperature which is 98.6°F/37°C). It tastes like apple cider. The vinegar brings across the mineral content from the apples, and the raw honey brings across the minerals in the nectar of the flowers. The honey must be pure and raw. It is believed to kill bacteria. The apple cider vinegar must also be pure and organic. The drink is a treatment and preventative of a variety of ailments and may help for overweight, chronic fatigue, chronic headaches, high blood pressure, blood sugar balance, dizziness, sore throat, mucus, muscle cramps, stuffy nose, sinusitis, hay fever, arthritis and even the common cold. It is important as the first drink in the morning upon awakening, as it will wash away any mucus residue which has accumulated in the digestive tract overnight. It may also cleanse the liver. During winter, fresh lemons (***not*** bottled lemon juice as this is preserved and extremely acidic), may be substituted for apple cider vinegar. Important: do not add lemon or lemon juice to hot liquid. Lemon is classified as an acid fruit but becomes alkaline in the system, however when it is added to hot liquid (or food), it will remain acid. **Please note** that the apple cider vinegar or lemon drink is recommended for an **alkaline system** and may aggravate existing imbalances, such as arthritis, in an already acid system. Follow the **Detox Diet (# 4)** or the **Acid/Alkaline Diet (# 3)** before drinking apple cider vinegar. Apple cider vinegar is versatile and can be used in many beneficial ways. Make a salad dressing with apple cider vinegar (or fresh lemon juice), olive oil, (optional) cottage cheese or plain yoghurt, garlic, parsley and other herbal seasonings.

BREAKFAST is the most important meal of the day for everybody regardless of age. It is the meal where the body is supplied with sufficient energy to cope with a large proportion of the day's demands. If inferior quality food is ingested, top performance can not be expected. Energy obtained from natural foods is not only required for brain, nerve and muscle function, but for the survival and functioning of every living cell in the body. A breakfast which contains protein, carbohydrates, fat, fiber, quality liquid, vitamins and minerals, is a bowl of fresh fruit, plain yogurt containing live cultures (optional), raw honey, nuts and seeds. This breakfast is filling, sustains blood sugar and provides many of the required nutrients.

CELERY & FENNEL: Celery is a natural diuretic and fennel is an appetite regulator. Both are useful for detoxification and weight control.

CEREALS (COLD): Eat only whole grain (which should be the first ingredient on the list). Avoid refined ingredients, milled grains, added sugars, chemicals and partially hydrogenated oils.

CEREALS (HOT): Oatmeal, oat bran, maize meal (grits) and sorghum (grass raised for grain) porridge are warming in winter. Adding cinnamon may destroy intestinal worms and parasites and taste especially nice with oatmeal. Avoid refined wheat-based porridge, as well as instant or microwave style. Eat whole grain that is the old fashioned cook-on-the- stove type.

CHEESE: All natural, naturally aged, made with milk from cows not treated with rBST (artificial growth hormone) in moderation. Unprocessed cheeses such as cottage and feta are less mucus forming.

Natural, uncolored cheeses should be eaten in moderation and processed cheese should be avoided.

COLD-PRESSED OILS: Extra virgin cold-pressed olive oil for salad dressings; organic virgin coconut oil for stir-fries. Use only cold-pressed vegetable and seed oils and avoid margarine and animal fats.

CINNAMON, CLOVE AND PUMPKIN SEEDS: Use these spices in cooking as their properties have the ability to destroy intestinal worms and parasites. Clove also destroys parasite eggs. Pumpkin seeds (Cucurbita pepo) have the ability to immobilize intestinal worms and aid in their expulsion.

DRINKING WITH MEALS: Drink either half an hour before or an hour after the meal. At least 70% of daily liquid intake should consist of water. Drink approximately 8 cups of **quality** liquid per day, e.g., filtered water, and fresh herbal tea. Drinking water should preferably be filtered. Certain drinking water may contain pesticides, insecticides, lead, chalk, herbicides, bacteria, lime, scale, slime, scum, asbestos and aluminum sulphate. Boiling water does not destroy chemicals. Chlorine, which kills bacteria in drinking water, may be harmful to us. Filtering water removes variable quantities of chlorine, bacteria, organic solids and some chemicals depending on which filtration method is used. Fresh fruit juices should be consumed in moderation as the sugar content is high. Commercial fruit juices should be avoided.

EGGS: Eat in moderation and preferably cage free eggs. Even if no health or blood vessel problems, do not eat more than 7 cage free eggs per week (1 per day) including baking and cooking. Purely in a humane effort, avoid eggs from chickens whose beaks have been mechanically trimmed (painful debeaking)

FRUIT & VEGETABLES: should be fresh and *in season*. Buy fresh in preference to frozen or canned. It is advisable to eat fruit in its season. In summer eat mostly fruit and in autumn eat mostly vegetables. In summer we perspire more, are involved in sport and outdoor activities and are generally more active due to the extended daylight hours and therefore use more energy. Nature has provided us with an abundance of fruit, which supplies pure liquids and energy, as well as cleansing our body. Summer fruits are especially juicy and refreshing, preventing dehydration. In autumn we are less active and need vegetables, which can be prepared in warm dishes such as soups, stews, casseroles and roasts. It is necessary to eat vegetables in autumn to prepare our bodies for the winter months. The vitamin and mineral contents obtained from vegetables prevent many winter illnesses.

Eat as much raw food as possible in the form of salads, vegetables and fruit. Chew well - digestion of carbohydrates begins with saliva. Melon fruit (watermelon, honeydew, sweet melon, cantaloupe) should be eaten alone (not with other fruit) as digestion is rapid and may take other undigested fruit through the system with it. Do not eat fruit with other cooked foods for the same reason - although, raw fruit and vegetables may be combined. Wait 30 to 60 minutes after eating fruit before eating other foods, but wait 3 to 4 hours after eating food which contains animal protein before eating fruit. This will prevent fermentation, as fatty foods could take up to 4 hours to digest.

At least 70% of daily food intake should consist of fruit, vegetables and salads which are alkaline forming. Cleanse your body by eating fruit for breakfast. Within 20 minutes the fruit has passed through the stomach into the intestines and is absorbed into the bloodstream, providing the body with energy. Most foods (including fruit and vegetables) contain proteins in the form of amino acids in varying degrees.

Keep natural foods whole where possible and avoid separation by peeling and juicing, as this deprives the food of their natural fibers.

Since natural foods are sprayed with insecticides, pesticides, fungicides and other poisons, which can be harmful to our systems if consumed, it is important to wash them (including nuts, seeds and grains) thoroughly. Certain contaminants are effectively diminished if the foods are washed in a basin of water with 2-3 tablespoons of apple cider vinegar. Commercial solutions obtainable at health food stores are also effective as they dispose of bacteria and large amounts of chemicals from sprays and fertilizers.

Natural foods supply vital energy obtained from the sun which is often depleted due to premature harvesting, cold storage, irradiation, artificial lighting in stores, packing and storage methods. This energy can be returned to fruits and vegetables to a large degree if placed in sunlight, as well as moonlight, for a couple of days before eating. Fresh produce should not be placed in direct sunlight as summer heat would scorch it. Placing fruits and vegetables in a basket, or suitable container, close to a window with ample sunlight is sufficient.

Dried fruit is a valuable snack, but must be eaten in moderation as it is high in concentrated sugar. Do not eat more dried fruit than would have been consumed if eating fresh fruit. Because the liquid has been evaporated from dried fruit, it is recommended to drink water to replace that lost liquid. Drinking water will prevent the dried fruit from absorbing too many fluids during the digestive process that is necessary for the actual process of digestion. Eat sun-dried fruit and avoid those with preservatives and other chemicals used to retain color or provide a shine.

GARLIC & PARSLEY: Garlic is a natural antibiotic and parsley detoxifies the body. Eat these, and other fresh herbs, often.

GRAINS: Wash thoroughly and numerous times (until clean) before cooking. Grains contain aflatoxins, which are micro toxins produced by fungus that colonize on crops.

HERBS: Grow your own (in the garden or in pots) and use them fresh - it's flavorful as well as healthy and medicinal.

HERBAL TEAS: Tea made with fresh herbs is healthier, more medicinal and tastes better than dried. If fresh is not available, then use dried herbs.

LEGUMES: Comprising of alfalfa, clover, peas, beans, lentils, lupins, mesquite, carob, and peanuts, are a good source of plant protein.

MEAT, POULTRY, PORK AND FISH: Meat and Poultry: Eat very sparingly, especially during summer and hot weather, as these proteins take longer to digest and cause other foods to ferment. It is healthier to concentrate on plant protein as excessive animal and dairy protein causes health problems. Because animals raised for the consumer industry cannot wash their foods they cannot avoid a long-term build-up of toxins, such as insecticides and pesticides in their bodies. They are also given antibiotics and growth hormones and a large quantity of these toxins and hormones are deposited in their tissue and are passed on to us. Animal protein is not a clean-burning fuel and we become what *they* eat, and the feed given to animals are NOT desirable. We would not feed to our pets what is fed to animals, yet we eat these animals in HUGE quantities. Through their flesh, their waste is deposited into our systems, which has to pass through our liver before *some* of it can be disposed of. Factory (and other) animals raised for the consumer industry are fed byproducts, which may contain any (or all) of the following: ground up feathers, hooves, beaks, dried blood, undeveloped chicken eggs, intestines, bone meal, offal, manure and poultry litter, fetal pigs, dead animals, same species dead meat and waste products. They are also fed distillers grains (from ethanol production), corn stover, plastic pellets (for roughage), drugs and chemicals.

If a more clean-burning fuel is desired, look for meat and animal products (milk, cheese, yoghurt, butter) that are certified organic and come from animals or poultry that are not factory farmed but free-range and cage-free. Consume beef from animals that are grass-fed (and very important) grass-finished (fattened) and not corn-finished. Pork should be pasture-raised, chickens should be cage-free and eggs should be from poultry that are cage-free.

Support local farmer's markets and buy their products but ensure they are organic. When buying from stores, select certified organic products and make certain eggs are from cage-fee hens on vegetarian feed (no animal byproducts) and their beaks have not been removed (debeaked).

In general, benefits from grass-fed meats are greater. The meat has more flavors and is leaner. High levels of natural antioxidant Conjugated Linoleic Acid (CLA) has more, and far greater health benefits than synthetic CLA.

<u>Mutton and lamb:</u> (as well as beef) are low in saturated fats and a much "cleaner burning fuel" if grass-fed and grass-finished (not corn fed or finished).

<u>Pork:</u> is known for its bacterial and parasitical content. People who consume pork should buy organic meat from pastured raised pigs, wash external bacterial off before cooking and cook at an internal heat of 160cF.

<u>Fish:</u> may come from polluted waters, contain mercury and parasites. Farm-raised fish (salmon, carp, tilapia, catfish and cod) contain **many** toxins obtained from their feed as well as growth hormones, antibiotics and other undesirable chemicals that pose health problems. Fish from deep ocean waters or certified wild, are healthier. The concern for how much mercury we take in depends greatly on how much fish we consume, as nearly all fish contain traces of mercury but some, definitely more than others. Fish low in mercury are salmon, shrimp, pollock, catfish, and canned light tuna - the latter depleted in nutrients due to the canning process. Wild fish from unpolluted waters are high in quality protein, omega-3 fatty acids and low in saturated fats.

MOLASSES is rich in potassium. It is a byproduct resulting from the process of refining sugar. The second extraction yields molasses as a thick, sweet liquid and the third extraction yields black-strap molasses. In the UK molasses is referred to as 'treacle' (Harry Potter's favorite dessert - treacle tart!). *Use in moderation,* as excess may (adversely) affect insulin production in the pancreas. Molasses is said to have many health benefits, but like most things, there are reports to the contrary as well.

MOLASSES (SORGHUM) Sorghum molasses (also referred to as sweet molasses) is not a true molasses. Sorghum is a grass but there are many different species used as grain for cereal, cane for sweet molasses, and distilled for alcohol in China. For sweet molasses (rich in iron and nutrients), natural juice is extracted and evaporated until the syrup is formed.

NUTS: Buy fresh nuts in their shells. The natural oils in shelled nuts are often rancid and may cause gas and bloating. Nuts in foil or vacuum packed packets may be slightly fresher than others, and is acceptable in moderation. Avoid flavored and spiced nuts as the flavorings may contain chemicals. Not more than 1 serving (or one hand full) of nuts should be eaten per day. Nuts should be raw (if possible) or roasted, well washed and well stored in air-tight containers.

REST AND RELAXATION: Do not over-exert your body. It is extremely important to rest one day of the week. Abstain from activities and shopping. Indulge in, not only a physical, but also a spiritual, mental and emotional rest. Our bodies are not designed to cope with stress 7 days a week, 12 months a year. For that reason we were given one day to rest. It is important to allow the vital organs of the body to rest. Renovating, gardening, shopping, playing sport may be fun but are not necessarily relaxing or resting, and we cannot enter a new week, week after week, exhausted. It is equally important to get enough sleep at night. The most important sleep is the 4 hours before and after midnight. 'Early to bed and early to rise' is a good rule to follow.

SALT: Use very sparingly - 50 - 100g per day. Use 'real' salts that are rich in minerals. Natural, unprocessed sea salt may have a slightly grey color as it is evaporated from sea water and is rich in minerals. Other options are vegetable salts and herb seasonings. Avoid chemical salts and seasonings, and those that contain anticaking agents.

SEEDS, DRIED FRUIT, SHELLED NUTS AND GRAINS should be washed before eating, as they are often covered in microscopic mold. Store in airtight containers and don't pre-wash all at once, only wash what you are about to eat.

SNACK FOOD: Should snacks be desired during the day, ensure they are **quality** snacks. The healthiest snacks to have are fresh fruit, salads (carrot and cucumber sticks, celery and almond butter, avocado) and vegetables (baked potato, corn on the cob). Sunflower seeds, nuts and sun dried fruit are also recommended. Other quality snacks (if not lactose intolerant) are live cultured plain yogurt sweetened with a little raw honey, raw brown sugar or stevia; rice salad consisting of brown rice and fresh diced vegetables, e.g., carrots, peas, corn, cucumber and celery. Use imagination, but **avoid** 'dead' and acid snacks such as cookies, cake, rusks, crackers, chips, candy, chocolates, bread, rolls, doughnuts and pastries. Eat food that will work and build the body, and not food that the body has to work to get out. In place of candy, eat fruit to satisfy sweet cravings.

SPROUTS are rich in vitamin B, C, E, minerals, protein and amino acids. Sprouts (especially wheat sprouts) should be from organic grains and seeds. Broccoli sprouts are extremely healthy.

SWEETENERS: Not all sweeteners are bad. There are natural sweeteners, and if taken in moderation, do not pose a problem.

Raw Brown Sugar: Avoid the sticky brown type. This is merely refined sugar with molasses added back. The best raw brown sugar is *Demerara cane sugar* which is obtained from fresh sugarcane juice that is washed and filtered, then heated to evaporate the water. The golden syrup is then crystallized. This is my choice of sweetener if used in moderation.

Raw Honey: kills bacteria and contains minerals. Do not confuse filtered or pure honey with raw honey. It must be unfiltered, unheated, raw honey. Do not put raw honey into liquids or food over 98.6°F/37°C degrees (body temperature), as heat will destroy valuable properties. Using raw honey in moderation does have certain medicinal benefits.

Maple syrup: Only use 100% pure, organic maple syrup as it contains vitamins and minerals. Use in moderation and *avoid artificial syrups!*

Stevia: is a Composite family herbal sweetener that has been used for centuries (pre-Columbian times). Controversy surrounds it as many people believe it to be safe with no ill effects while 'some people' would like many people to think it an "unsafe food additive", suggesting it is a type of narcotic. I have seen many children and adults get 'high' on white sugar on a daily basis, but never on stevia. It is now marketed as a dietary supplement.

THICKENERS: For gravy, soups, casseroles, etc. Use natural ingredients such as cornstarch, potato flour or rice flour, etc.

WATER: Water from faucets should contain the same energy as that from a stream, but pollution, chemicals and transportation through dirty, rusty pipes result in water depleted in natural minerals and energy. Leaving filtered water in a clear glass jug in the sun for a number of hours will restore some of the lost energy.

WHOLE GRAIN CRACKERS: Rye crackers and rice cakes can be eaten in moderation as snacks, but it is more beneficial to avoid these. Wheat products, rye crackers and rice cakes are termed 'dry' foods. Our system requires natural 'wet' foods and hence we will benefit more from natural foods such as fruit, salads, vegetables, beans, brown rice, legumes, nuts, seeds and all other nature-made foods. Man-made foods may cause imbalances which lead to dis-ease and later disease. Avoid refined crackers as they may contain partially hydrogenated oils.

WHOLE FOODS SEPARATED: I am not a huge supporter of separating natural foods and try to keep this to a minimum. Separating natural foods would be, for example, eating only egg-white omelettes, or eating molasses, or drinking orange juice. I prefer eating the 'whole' food i.e. omelettes with egg-white and yolk combined; or eating a whole orange rather than separate the fruit from the juice, and drinking the juice only. Rightfully so, egg yolks do contain cholesterol but nature places the correct amount of lecithin in egg-white to balance the whole egg. Drinking orange juice is concentrated sugar, which reaches the pancreas more rapidly than when eating the whole orange. By eating the whole fruit, it provides much needed fiber and nutrients that aid in preventing a concentrated sugar impact on the pancreas.

WHOLE CEREALS: Eat granola/muesli, oatmeal, and oat bran. Avoid wheat, wheat bran and wheat containing products as much as possible.

WHOLE GRAINS: A whole grain is termed thus when three parts (bran, germ and endosperm) are present. Whole grains are packed with nutrients and eating whole grains may lower the risk of chronic diseases. Brown and wild rice is good for the nervous system. Barley keeps colds away. Corn is a good source of fiber. The list is vast. **Whole grains should be organic and not genetically modified.** A few good whole grains are: amaranth, barley, brown and wild rice, bulgur or cracked wheat, couscous, flaxseed (classified as grain or seed), millet (cereal grain), oats, popcorn, quinoa, rye, sorghum (grass grain) spelt, wheat, and wheat berries (whole grain).

WHEAT: For more information, refer to "FOODS TO AVOID" I do not endorse products as companies change and ingredients alter but I do willingly promote Wheat Montana. This wheat is as nature intended. It is 100% whole wheat, GMO and chemical free, nothing removed and nothing added. Bronze Chief and Prairie Gold are the two whole wheat flour I recommend for making anything where flour is required. I wish more companies would produce grains the same as Wheat Montana do.

YOGURT: Live cultured yogurt replaces friendly bacteria in the colon. It is easy to make (see recipe for YOGURT) or buy unflavored commercial yogurt made with live AB cultures. If desired, sweeten with a little raw honey or stevia, and add fresh fruit - avoid artificially sweetened, flavored and colored yoghurt as well as those that are soy based.

FOODS TO AVOID

Avoid foods that are bad quality acids (i.e. refined and chemical man-made foods) as these lead to a build up of toxins within the body, which in turn, become disease forming.

ALCOHOL is not recommended and should be avoided. If unable to abstain, consumption should be in very small quantities, preferably additive-free and made from organically grown ingredients. Drink spirits with water (plain or naturally carbonated) and avoid chemical, carbonated sodas. Search for wines, spirits and beers that are low in alcohol contents, made with pure ingredients, are not chemically enhanced, and do not contain preservatives.

ALUMINUM COOKING UTENSILS: Use surgical stainless steel or glass cookware. Do not cook or store food in aluminum containers.

CHOCOLATE, COCOA AND OTHER FLAVORED MILK DRINKS: Avoid formulas for hot and cold drinks mixed with milk or water as they are acid forming, contain refined sugar and many other chemicals such as flavorings and colorings.

CRUMBED & PARTIALLY PREPARED COMMERCIAL FROZEN FOODS contain preservatives and flavorings. Crumbed foods are treated with a chemical, which assist the crumbs to adhere to the surface.

DECAFFEINATED COFFEE still contains two stimulants, theobromine and theophylline. Drinking tea or coffee at mealtimes may inhibit both iron and zinc absorption.

CARBONATED (SODA POP) & CORDIAL COLD DRINKS are pure chemical drinks and do nothing but harm the system. If a carbonated drink is desired, have carbonated 100% pure fruit juice *in moderation*. 100% pure fruit juices, which are not carbonated are very concentrated and contain large amounts of sugar so need to be diluted with water and consumed in moderation. In addition, these juices are pasteurized (boiled), which makes them acidic. There has been controversy regarding the possible disadvantages of containers lined with aluminum foil. Avoid all concentrated cordials drinks, which are mixed with water or carbonated water; as well as commercial concentrated 'fresh' orange, grapefruit or other concentrated juices. Avoid commercial drinks that are dairy and fruit; or dairy and chocolate; or other flavor mixtures. Avoid all drinks that are not 100% pure fruit juice, and contain colorings, flavorings, additives and preservatives. **We become what we eat and drink.** Nature gave us water to drink and fruit to eat.

CHOCOLATES: Although very tasty, we eat too many. Statistics in England has revealed that on average people consume 8kgs/17.6lbs of chocolates per annum per person. It has been suggested that pure organic chocolate contains the highest antioxidant properties, but this is only so if not adulterated with refined sugars, dairy, flavorings and other chemical fillers.

ICE CREAM: Today, many more organic and pure ingredient ice creams are obtainable which may be enjoyed *in moderation*. Be mindful of cheap ice creams that have substituted natural ingredients with artificial and chemical ingredients, as these may be harmful to our systems.

The following is an extract from the book *"Reflexology - a Practical Introduction"* written by Inge Dougans.

These are some additives found in certain commercially produced ice cream:

Piperonal: used in place of vanilla - is a chemical used to treat lice.

Diethyl glucol: cheap chemical used as an emulsifier instead of eggs. Also used in antifreeze and paint removers.

Butyraldehyde: used in nut flavored ice cream - one of the ingredients in rubber cement.

Amyl acetate: used for banana flavor - is also an oil paint solvent.

Ethyl acetate: used for pineapple flavor - also used as a cleaner for leather and textiles.

Aldehyde C17: flavors cherry ice cream - an inflammable liquid used in aniline dyes, plastic and rubber.

LEFT-OVER FOOD: I am frequently asked my opinion on left-over food. Strictly speaking, sufficient food should be prepared and consumed at a sitting without any being left over. Often, this is unavoidable and we have nutritious food in excess. It is a waste to discard it. Seal left over food in airtight containers and refrigerate no longer than 24 hours. Use as quickly as possible.

I would rather a person take a small container of nutritious home prepared food to work the next day than a nutrient depleted sandwich, crackers, cookies or any other refined convenience food.

PLASTIC CONTAINERS AND WRAP: The next question I am asked is "which containers are suitable for storing food?" There are many wonderful airtight plastic containers available, designed to serve this purpose. I do need to caution against the effects chemicals in plastic, polystyrene and other containers may have on our health. We use plastic on a daily basis - we drink out of it, eat off it and store substances in it. Furthermore, we purchase many of our consumables wrapped or packaged in it. Research has us asking "is it safe to store our foods in it - can chemicals found in plastic transfer to our food and pose a safety risk for us and our children?" Baby bottles have been an enormous concern as a chemical in the plastic called Bisphenol-A (BPA) was found, during tests conducted, to seep out in small amounts. Experts have warned that the effects of BPA could be as far-reaching as causing developmental disruption affecting behavior, intelligence and learning ability. It could store in the body and years later cause infertility. Colored and opaque baby bottles contain less harmful levels of BPA. If possible find out, before purchasing items, if they contain BPA by contacting the manufacturer.

A team of researchers from the University of Missouri-Columbia and North Carolina State University reported that BPA (a compound originally made as a chemical estrogen), now used as a 'building block' for the production of polycarbonate plastic products which include storage containers, tin can linings, babies bottles and certain toys, produce premature puberty, changes in growth and reproductive abnormalities as well as weight gain.

Babies are not the only ones at risk. DEHA is a chemical used to make certain plastic wraps soft and clingy. This chemical has the ability to seep out of the wrap in small amounts and penetrate all fatty products such as milk, butter, yogurt, cheese, meat and any other fat-containing substance. Tests revealed that it took as little as half an hour for seepage to occur.

Certain plastic containers do not contain DEHA and can not be included in this group. Glass containers, although not as durable, are far safer to use for storage.

MARGARINE contains colorings and may contain nickel (a toxic metal) as a catalyst to convert it to hard fat. This tends to accumulate in the liver, as we cannot metabolize it completely. Rather use butter in moderation. For baking and cooking, cold-pressed vegetable oils, such olive oil or organic coconut oil, are preferable.

NICOTINE is a poisonous alkaloid contained in tobacco and is known to cause many different cancers. Smoking also causes hardening of the arteries, large and small. Tiny arteries carrying valuable nutrients to the eyes and ears are affected leading to bad eyesight and deafness.

PEANUTS: Eat raw, unsalted peanuts in moderation, but roast or wash in apple cider vinegar water before eating to clean off mold. Peanuts are a 'social' carcinogen because of aflatoxins found in moldy foods. (A carcinogen is a substance which causes cancerous changes in cells.) Other social carcinogens are alcoholic drinks; over-eating (causing obesity); a high saturated fat or high refined sugar, low fiber diet; tobacco smoking; ultraviolet light; pesticides; ionizing radiation; nitrates in preserved meats; nitrates in preservatives and water supplies; azo food dyes.

PRESERVATIVES, COLORINGS, ARTIFICIAL FLAVORINGS, ADDITIVES: Read labels. We are not designed to consume chemical cocktails, as these collect in our system and contribute to ill health. Avoid packet soups, sauces, marinades and other convenience foods laced with chemicals.

REFINED FOODS: White flour, white rice and white sugar. All refined foods are 'dead' foods, which are depleted in nutrients. Eat 'live' foods which are nutrient rich, such as fruit, salads and vegetables. **Remember that you are what you eat, and what you eat will become you**!

SMOKED AND PROCESSED FOODS as well as CANNED, BOTTLED AND PACKAGED FOODS should not take the place of fresh food. Fresh is best; if there are no options, then revert to frozen before canned.

SOY AND SOY PRODUCTS: It is estimated that more than 90% of soy in the USA is genetically modified (GM). Many ailments caused by the consumption of soy are misdiagnosed, and consequently 'mistreated'. Unfermented soy may cause fermentation in the digestive system resulting in gas and bloating and may aggravate conditions such as eczema and psoriasis. Soy-based baby milk may cause diaper rash and colic in babies. Soy products are processed foods, which are acidic and 'dead' and no different from other processed foods. GM-soy is widely used in the food industry and can be found in cereals, processed meat, bread, fast foods, pasta, spreads, and many other products. The actions of soy phytoestrogens in the body have been linked to breast cancer, thyroid imbalances, and many other ailments.

Fermented soy (miso, paste, sauces, tamari, tempeh, natto, fermented tofu, and fermented soy milk) has more health benefits than unfermented soy (unfermented tofu, unfermented soy milk).

Care needs to be taken when purchasing soy beans and products, as most soy beans are genetically modified. I am totally against consuming soy as I have seen, for over twenty years, its effects on the human body i.e. skin rashes, itches, scalp problems. My advice to those using soy is to buy fermented soy and use in extreme moderation. For more information on GE foods, refer to Chapter 16.

SUGAR AND SUGAR PRODUCTS:

Agave: mainly Mexican in origin, looks like an Aloe plant (but is not Aloe or cacti); it is related more to the lily families. Agave nectar (or syrup), which is released from the base of the flower stalk, is used as a sweetener after its refining process. Its claim to fame is that it is suppose to be the lowest on the glycemic index, and when certain parts of the plant are fermented and distilled, Tequila spirits are produced.

I personally am not a fan of agave and do not promote it as an acceptable sweetener, as it is a highly refined form of fructose as a result of it refining process.

Jams, cookies, candy, pastries, soda pop, cakes, ice cream, etc.: Research estimates that we consume an excess of 2.2 lbs/1 kg sugar per week in 'hidden' sugar such as sweeteners and preservatives used in canned, packaged and bottled foods. Refined sugar may be carcinogenic, and may increase the incidence of cancer. If sugar is used, the best kind is *Demerara cane sugar* derived from evaporated cane juice. Avoid the sticky, caramel brown sugar.

SUGAR SUBSTITUTES: To my knowledge, there is no ‘good’ artificial sweetener. Rather use raw brown sugar (evaporated cane juice), raw honey or stevia sparingly. I do not encourage or recommend sweeteners at all but for those who insist, I can only recommend that they educate themselves as to the dangers of artificial sweeteners and use them with extreme caution. Many diseases and side-effects have been attributed to the use of these, and information is available on a large scale through the Internet. The following symptoms have been linked to the use of aspartame: headaches, dizziness, mood swings, vomiting or nausea, abdominal pain or cramps, vision disturbances, diarrhea, seizures or convulsions, memory loss, fatigue, weakness, neurological imbalances, rash, sleep problems, hives, change in heart rate, itching of the skin, numbness, tingling, local swelling, inactivity and breathing difficulties.

TEA & COFFEE: These are acid forming, stimulating and contain substances which may harm various organs and impair their functions. Herbal coffee substitutes are healthier than ordinary coffee, but they are still acid forming and should be consumed in moderation. Avoid flavored teas and rather have herbal teas, which have health benefits.

WHEAT: Avoid bread, pasta, cookies, pizza, pastries, and all other wheat products. One reasons is that it has a high content of glutelins and promaline (protein types) causing sensitivities which aggravate allergies such as sinus, asthma, hay fever, eczema and psoriasis. It further causes digestive discomforts such as indigestion, irritable bowel, gas, bloating, spastic colon, and can lead to constipation, which in a chronic state can cause serious health threatening diseases.

Wheat products can be replaced with, for example, granola/muesli, maize meal (grits), rice cakes or rye crackers. Those who really can't do without wheat, should limit their wheat intake to once a day only, e.g., if they have toast or wheat cereal at breakfast, don't have sandwiches for lunch and pasta or pizza at dinner; if they have sandwiches or pizza at lunch, avoid further wheat products at breakfast and dinner; and if they know they are going to have pasta for dinner, don't have wheat products for breakfast, lunch and snacks. Should they be invited to a festivity or celebration and they know they are going to have cake, cookies or similar 'treats', avoid wheat at all other meals and possibly for a few days thereafter.

I strongly recommend that a 4-day rotation is adopted with all grains. This means that a grain is eaten only once a day (at one meal) and then not again for at least 4 days. This will not cause the immune system to over react as the body will not be 'invaded' multiple times per day by one food type. For this very same reason, Nature has given us different foods produced in different seasons. Because of imports and refrigeration, we no longer eat 'in season' and by eating the same foods daily, multiple times per day, we excite an immune response and cause the body to over react, activating white blood cells, resulting in allergies and food sensitivities.

There are many wonderful, nutritious **organic** whole grains that can, and should, be brought into our diets: amaranth, barley, brown and wild rice, bulgur or cracked wheat, couscous, flaxseed (technically not a grain), millet (cereal grain), oats, popcorn, quinoa, rye, sorghum (grass grain), spelt, wheat, and wheat berries (whole grain). **Always make certain grains are not genetically modified (genetically engineered)!**

80-90% of health complaints relate to wheat sensitivities due to:

1) **The immune system** responding to an over exposure to wheat. White blood cells are activated and allergies result.

2) **Genetic engineering** of wheat uses a host of chemicals to change the DNA structure from long grain to short grain to make it possible to grow in different countries. The wheat now contains double the chromosomes needed. This renders wheat incompatible with human enzymes and causes digestive complications. For more information, refer to Chapter 16.

3) **Chemicals and pesticides** sprayed on wheat to prevent destruction by wheat lice and other pests. It is sprayed or fumigated further when it is stored in silos, and these chemicals are carried forward through the milling process and ingested by us. We are unable to digest these (carcinogenic) chemicals and they cause adverse effects, such as sensitivities and allergies in our bodies.

4) **Aflatoxins:** toxins produced by the bacterium *aspergillus flavus*. The bacterium develops in mildew which grows inside grain silos. Found in peanuts, bread, oil and margarine produced from certain seeds; meat from animals fed on contaminated wheat or corn; poultry, milk and eggs, from wheat and corn fed animals. Aflatoxins cause

cirrhosis and liver cancer. This is one reason why it is advisable to buy wheat and gluten free products, and animal protein and products from grass fed (and grass finished) livestock.

Wheat and flour from Wheat Montana do not qualify in this category as their grains are the purest I have encountered. I fully support their products i.e. Bronze Chief and Prairie Gold. As previously mentioned (but it deserves reiteration) Wheat Montana is as nature intended. It is 100% whole wheat, GMO and chemical free, nothing removed and nothing added. I avoid eating bread and wheat products, but if I am going to use wheat flour for anything, Bronze Chief and Prairie Gold are the two whole wheat flour I use.

YOGURT: Avoid flavored and colored yogurt. Eat unflavored yogurt and flavor with fresh fruit and nuts.

CONCLUSION

Many of our foods are inferior and contain chemicals that are harmful to our systems, causing pain and discomfort, which financially costs thousands in medical bills and often results in unnecessary operations. Yet many manufacturers produce these foods and advertise them in a fashion that leads us to believe we are purchasing top quality, healthy products.

We need to become more informed, more aware, and more concerned with what we are putting into our bodies, as well as our children's bodies. We need to take a stand with the foods we purchase and demand better quality as well as better control. Why must butter have colorings and flavoring or salt added? Why can we not buy 100% natural butter? This is merely one example!

If every person with a wheat sensitivity stopped buying wheat-based products, probably 90% of the population would be involved, and manufacturers as well as bakers of wheat products would soon turn to an alternative source, or quality flour. They could use non-genetically modified wheat, rice, corn, rye, barley or the many other whole grains available for flour. This in turn would force the farmers who grow genetically modified (GM) wheat to investigate the problem and correct it where possible and switch back to growing non-genetically modified grains.

The problem is, GM grains and ingredients are less expensive than its non-GM counterpart. For this reason, there will always be manufacturers producing 'cheap' products made with GM ingredients. There will always be people buying these 'cheap' products. This encourages the competitive market to produce more cheap foods using cheap ingredients. When healthy foods are manufactured with non-GM ingredients, the price increases and consumer weigh up monetary benefits before health benefits - not realizing that pennies saved today will cost thousands of dollars later in medical bills.

Consumers in the European Union (EU) and Japan (and many in Australia and New Zealand) demand more exposure to GM foods by way of product labeling. This allows individuals to make their choices. I sincerely hope people will become more informed about what is in their foods and make healthier choices. Eating good, natural food should be a daily activity and become a lifestyle, and not a short-term diet.

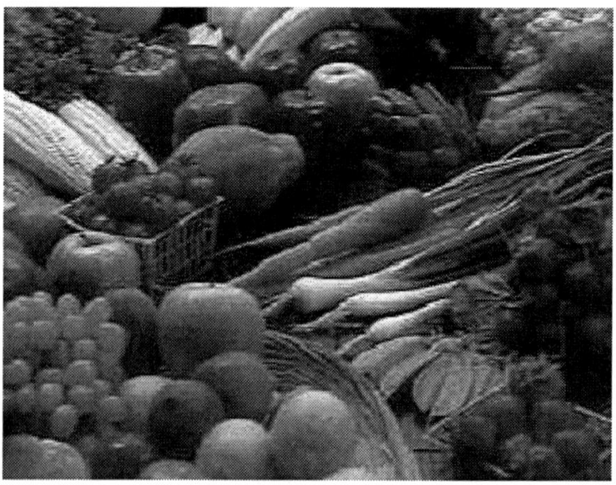

KEY TO GOOD HEALTH

The following simple rules are the key to good health:

- ❑ Eat meat and poultry as little as possible. Animal protein is more compatible with our bodies in winter than summer.
- ❑ Eat fish that are certified wild, or from deep ocean waters.
- ❑ Eat natural foods such as vegetables (raw or cooked), fruit, herbs, nuts, seeds and whole-grains. These are rich in nutrients, fiber, vitamins and minerals.
- ❑ Eat natural foods fresh and in its season.
- ❑ Eat natural foods that are organic, and not genetically modified.
- ❑ Drink water as your main liquid intake. Herbal teas should be consumed in moderation. Fresh vegetable or fruit juices should be used to supply nutrients when meals cannot be eaten.
- ❑ Avoid all chemical hot drinks including tea and coffee.
- ❑ Avoid all chemical cold drinks including ice cold water. Liquids vastly higher or lower than body temperature cause an imbalance in the body's temperature homeostasis.
- ❑ Avoid drinking with meals as this dilutes digestive juices, prolonging the process of digestion.
- ❑ Avoid alcohol - there is no such thing as moderation!
- ❑ Avoid nicotine.
- ❑ Avoid man-made and genetically engineered foods. Only nature produces perfect food.

*Everything you consume will eventually become **you**. It forms part of your skin, nails, hair, brain function, hormonal excretions. Choose wisely, as **you are what you eat**... "therefore, let food be thy medicine"*

CHAPTER 3
PREGNANCY

LIFESTYLE BEFORE CONCEPTION: It is very important that both the male and female detoxify and adopt a healthy lifestyle long before the baby is conceived, so that **both** their bodies are free of toxins, and they are able to produce and develop a healthy baby. Health does not start with the onset of pregnancy, but the pregnancy depends entirely on how healthy both were at the time (as well as before) conception. A baby is only as healthy as the present condition of the sperm and the ovum. There is no law that guarantees a healthy baby once fertilization has taken place. The child is formed from half the mother and half the father's genes. If one or both parents live unhealthily or fill their systems with refined, processed or chemical foods, the baby can only be formed (and nourished) from the nutrients existing in their systems. Think about it - *it takes two to make a healthy child.*

As important is the mother's diet during pregnancy, as this will affect her health as well as the baby's. During the first four months, protein is needed for growth and development, keeping in mind that plant protein is healthier than animal protein. To combat tiredness experienced by expectant mothers, natural foods are imperative as they provide energy, vitamins and minerals. Although glucose is necessary for brain development, refined sugars and starches should be avoided and substituted with fruit, root vegetables, and legumes.

Natural foods will prevent weight gain, which is a health hazard and can lead to varicose veins, hemorrhoids, depression, and numerous other pregnancy related dis-eases. Excess weight can also cause complications during the final stages of pregnancy and labor. It is very difficult to lose excess weight after the birth and this can lead to depression.

Equally dangerous is malnutrition resulting from food deprivation due to fear of obesity. This could result in impaired growth and development for the baby as well as difficulties with breast-feeding.

If one parent has a history of allergies, the baby has a 40% chance of being an allergy sufferer, but if both parents have a history of allergies, the baby has a 60% chance of being an allergy sufferer. This can be avoided and the statistics reduced drastically if the mother avoids wheat and soy, as well as wheat and soy products during pregnancy. Should the mother have a desire for wheat in the form of bread or pasta, she could eat wheat-free rye bread, cornbread, potato bread, rice or corn pasta and many of the other wheat free products available from health food stores and similar stores.

Ensure that all grains used as ingredients are not genetically modified or refined. Keep in mind that a pure rye bread is not readily available, as most rye breads still contains 50% or more wheat, and are thus not recommended. 100% rye crackers are a good substitute to use in place of wheat crackers. These can be used as "open-faced" sandwiches with almond butter; hummus; cottage or Swiss cheese, tomatoes and cucumber; boiled egg or tuna with homemade mayonnaise or store-bought grapeseed vegan-'naise' (obtainable from health food stores).

Pregnant women need a good natural multi-vitamin and mineral supplement (made with 'live' ingredients) with added folic acid, vitamin B6, calcium and iron. These nutrients are readily obtained from cottage cheese, natural yogurt, whole grains and green leafy vegetables, and other natural foods. Vitamin B6 and ginger tea are reputed to minimize morning sickness. Eating natural foods with dietary fiber, vitamins and minerals is the only way to ensure a healthy pregnancy and baby, limiting obesity, stretch marks, constipation, varicose veins, hemorrhoids and a host of other complaints.

To prevent over-sized and later sagging breasts with stretch marks, it is recommended that the pregnant mother wear a good cotton bra day and night. It is important she **sleeps with the bra on** from the early stages of pregnancy (as soon as the breasts start enlarging), until at least three months ***after*** she has stopped breast-feeding.

DIET # 1: PREGNANCY

Daily nutrition largely determines the quality of pregnancy as well as labor and quick recovery, regaining strength and the ability to cope with the new demand.

Protein, wheat and dairy should only be natural, organic, non-genetically modified (non-GM) products that are hormone, antibiotic, and chemical free. Fish should be wild, or from deep ocean waters.

GRAINS: All foods containing wheat should be replaced with non-GM whole grain foods such as amaranth, barley, brown and wild rice, bulgur or cracked wheat, couscous, flaxseed (an ancient grain), millet (cereal grain), oats, popcorn, quinoa, rye, sorghum (grass grain), spelt and organic wheat.

Implement a 4-day rotation with all grains. Eat one grain only once a day (at one meal) and then not again for at least 4 days. This will not cause the immune system to over react as the body will not be 'invaded' multiple times per day by one food type. For this reason, nature has given us different foods produced in different seasons. Because of imports and refrigeration, we no longer eat 'in season' and by eating the same foods daily, multiple times per day, we excite an immune response and cause the body to over react, activating white blood cells, resulting in allergies and food sensitivities. On the 4-day rotation, legumes can be eaten at other meals where grain is not eaten.

PLANT PROTEIN: is nutrient rich and strengthens the immune system. These include foods such as: nuts, seeds and legumes.

LEGUMES: the following foods are legumes: alfalfa, clover, peas, beans, lentils, lupins, mesquite, carob, and peanuts. Apart from being a good source of fiber, legumes maintains sustained blood sugar, assists in preventing cholesterol and supplies valuable minerals such as folic acid, iron, magnesium and copper.

OILS AND FATS: These are equally important during pregnancy and should be obtained from cold-pressed fruits (olive, avocado), nuts (almond, walnut, hazelnut), seeds (sunflower, sesame, grapeseed, pumpkin, chia), grains (wheat germ). Fresh avocado is an excellent source of vegetable protein and fat, which is needed for the building and repair of cell membranes, healthy nervous system and transportation of fat-soluble vitamins.

FISH: should be wild and from deep ocean waters. Avoid farmed fish as their growth hormones and steroids are definitely not needed during pregnancy when natural hormonal levels are elevated anyway.

DAIRY: If milk tolerant, eat natural uncolored cheese (in moderation), as well as feta and cottage cheese, but avoid 'moldy' and processed cheese.

MEAT AND POULTRY: Lamb, beef, pork and poultry should be organic, grass-fed, grass-finished, pasture-raised and cage-free.

PROTEIN: 'pure' (organic) plant and animal protein is important during pregnancy as it is used for building and repair and the development of new cells. Pregnant women's blood volume increases during pregnancy and protein is needed for this function.

The diet should consist of fruit, salads, vegetables, sprouts, nuts (almonds are alkaline forming) seeds, plant protein, organic animal protein (optional), organic whole grains, legumes, cold pressed oils (e.g. olive), and quality sweeteners such as stevia, raw honey or raw brown sugar, in moderation.

HONEY: is an excellent food source as well as food supplement and prevents fermentation in the gastro-intestinal tract. It is recommended to have two teaspoons a day in the diet as either a sweetener, direct from the spoon, or on rye crackers, cornbread or rice cake. Honey is quickly absorbed into the blood stream. It contains important elements for forming new blood and will aid the fetus in building a good nervous system. Honey is a mild laxative and will prevent constipation as well as being a sedative.

CONSTIPATION: avoid constipation by reducing 'dry' foods (bread, pasta, crackers) and drink two glasses of water every morning, afternoon and evening. Cold pressed olive oil eaten with salads will further reduce the risk of constipation.

MORNING SICKNESS: This varies with women and can be mild or severe. Increased hormonal levels, especially progesterone and estrogen, may be huge contributors. Rather than eating refined crackers, drinking fresh ginger tea with raw honey is much healthier. This is made by steeping (soaking) 3 to 6 slices ginger (depending on desired strength) in a cup of hot water for 5 minutes. Sweeten to taste with a little raw honey. Sip slowly and enjoy twice daily.

BALANCED MEAL: Daily consumption should include at least 3 fruits, a bowl of salad, 2 raw or cooked vegetables, a hand full of raw nuts (almonds), organic protein, whole grain, and water to drink. Quantities will vary according to mass. To obtain a better balance of acid and alkaline foods, the daily intake should consist of 70%-80% alkaline and 20%-30% acid forming foods, summarized as follows:

Alkaline foods: vegetables; vegetable juices; alkaline fruits; sprouts, natural herbs and herbal tea; nuts (almonds); seeds (sunflower, pumpkin, chia seeds)

Acid foods: organic protein; organic whole grains; acid fruits, legumes, nuts and certain sweeteners (raw brown sugar, raw honey, stevia).

Avoid citrus fruit and citrus juices when out of season - eat only when fresh and in season and avoid again towards the end of the citrus season as these products rapidly become too acidic, especially when they have been stored. Enjoy grapes, apples and cranberries when in season. The latter will prevent bladder infections. Dilute grape juice with water to reduce sugar content.

AVOID: ordinary tea; coffee (even decaffeinated); nicotine; alcohol; protein and dairy that is not organic; all carbonated drinks including diet drinks; cordials and all drinks not 100% pure; sugar and sugar products (candy, chocolates, cakes, cookies, jams); sugar substitutes; refined food (bread, pasta, pizza, pastries); preservatives; coloring and artificial flavorings; additives; chemical ice cream; commercial colored and flavored yogurt; margarine (eat organic butter in moderation); smoked and processed meats or foods; canned foods; aluminum cooking utensils; drinking with meals; cooked or fried tomatoes (eat only raw tomatoes as heat alters the pH balance); crumbed/breaded and partly prepared foods; commercial frozen foods. Concentrate on whole and fresh foods such as fruit, salads, vegetables, sprouts, nuts, seeds, brown or wild rice, beans, lentils and other pulses and whole grains.

APPLE CIDER VINEGAR: Dr. Jarvis from Vermont, USA, who is an expert on apple cider vinegar, said in his book *"Folk Medicine"* that an expectant mother who makes the effort to eat natural, pure and whole foods daily (and cuts out junk), can expect to give birth to a baby who has a lot of hair on its head; has fingernails that are strong and long enough to cut; has a good digestive system and eliminates without problems; has a good face width with a well-shaped jaw enabling teeth to come out uncrowded; is mentally bright and has a strong muscular system. The baby will be able to lift its head up off the pillow unaided before it is a week old and as it grows, it will have good brain-muscle coordination, strong teeth and no allergies.

An expectant mother should take the following throughout her pregnancy: On rising, one teaspoon apple cider vinegar in a glass of water (this prevents or clears up morning sickness as well). At one other meal during the day, two teaspoons apple cider vinegar and two teaspoons raw honey in water.

BREAST MILK: Breast is best for baby but remember that the milk is only produced from the raw materials provided in the form of food and liquids placed within it the digestive system. Alcohol and drugs go to the baby by way of breast milk. Inferior diets will produce inferior milk and will directly affect the development of the baby. For this reason it is imperative that a good, natural, nutrient rich diet is followed. During pregnancy, the food eaten will lay the foundation for the eventual milk production when the baby is born. **You are what you eat and the baby will become what you eat as well.**

CHAPTER 4
BABIES

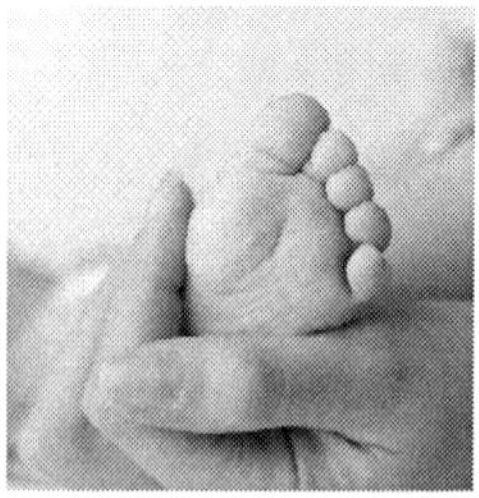

As mentioned in the previous chapter - breast is best! Breast milk is conveniently packaged, kept sterile, maintained at the correct temperature and ready to serve - any time - any place. Although the breast is best, it must be kept in mind that it is only as good as the mother's diet. The food the mother eats eventually becomes her blood from which the milk is produced. **Breast milk is formulated by nature and is the most ideal food for the infant's immature digestive system, reducing gastric problems and reactions to allergies.**

Most valuable is the colostrum secreted for approximately three days after the birth. Continuing for a further few days, breast milk consists of valuable colostrum which contains the mother's antibodies needed to protect the infant against gastroenteritis and many other diseases. To ensure successful feeding with high quality breast milk, it is required of the lactating mother to continue with a nutritious diet and adequate intake of quality liquids, such as herbal teas and filtered water. Pure fruit juices must be diluted with filtered water and taken *in moderation.*

Babies should be exclusively breast fed until their teeth appear, which under normal circumstances may take four to six months. There is no need for water, as the first part of the breast milk quenches the thirst and the second part contains the 'cream', which feeds the baby. A calendar cannot tell when the baby is ready for solid foods but nature can - by producing their teeth. Solid foods in a pureed form should be introduced when the baby has started teething. Avoid cereals as they are refined and lead to allergies, and concentrate on pureeing natural fruit, vegetables and grains, introducing new foods gradually. Introducing new foods every two to three days will avoid allergies, or afford the opportunity to distinguish allergy-causing foods.

Babies should be prepared for solid foods by being gradually introduced to the smell, feel and taste of food from the age of four months onward. This does not mean feeding them, but merely introducing them to the foods. The brain needs to register new smells, tastes and touch, and this is done by allowing the child to taste what is being eaten by dipping a clean finger into natural food and then running it through their mouth. When babies are ready to sit in a feeding chair, they should be allowed to touch and 'feel' food. Be less concerned about how clean baby must remain and focus more on the much needed 'discovery' experience. When they teethe, allow them to suck on solid foods such as a chicken drum stick or lamb chop bone, carrot, cucumber, apple, celery stick etc., taking care that the food does not break off and choke the child. Do **not** give them cookies, toast, crackers and other wheat cereals or foods that are refined and depleted of nutrients, and have very little nutritional value but only serve to 'fill' the baby. Sugar in refined cereals and foods will further lower the baby's immune system and affect their development.

Babies have taste buds, and when feeding them the food should be tasty and desirable, but avoid adding salt, butter and sugar. Root vegetables such as sweet potatoes or yams are naturally sweet and add a pleasant taste to foods. Pureed fruit and natural yogurt (if no milk allergies) is light and easily digested. For breakfast, thinly made porridge or hot cereals such as maize meal (grits) and oatmeal may be given, but avoid refined, manufactured cereals, as these have very little nutritional value and could contribute to allergies or food sensitivities. The only cereals I recommend are made from fresh, organic, untreated and unsprayed grains, such as oats, barley and rice. The grains are cooked into a cereal cream by boiling thoroughly with water and then liquidizing it or pressing it through a food mill, producing a smooth paste. As the baby grows, vegetables may be added and cooked with the grains. Grains pass through the 'milk stage' when ripening, and contain a rich milky liquid, which hardens to become the core of the grain. Boiled with sufficient water, the core becomes creamy again, and rice, barley and oats are particularly abundant with this cream which provides a complete balanced food for humans - perfect for the infant's transition from breast milk to solids. Cereal creams can also be prepared from grains finely ground into flour and 1 part flour in 10 - 15 parts water, boiled for 20 minutes. For added nutrients, seeds and later beans could be ground with the grains. The concept of nutritious cereal creams was lost when they were replaced with refined commercial cereals, popular for their convenience. Mothers are unaware that these foods lack valuable nutrients and thus inhibit the development of the immune system, slowly leading to health imbalances.

Cereal milks of high dilution are recommended where a mother has breast feeding problems, as these are far more natural than formulas. In this situation, water from cooked vegetables for the very young (2 to 4 months) and thinly pureed vegetables for the babies 4 to 6 months, could be added to ensure sufficient vitamin and mineral intake. Cereal milks can become progressively thicker as the baby grows, and can then be introduced as cereal creams with pureed vegetables.

After 8 months, or when they are ready to chew (using the number of teeth they have as a guideline), whole grains can be cooked, but with a larger proportion of water than would be used when preparing for adults. Mashed, rather than pureed, vegetables should be added to the grains.

If babies are introduced to ice cream, chocolates, cookies and other sweet foods, the taste will register in the brain and a sweet-toothed child will grow up being fussy and picky with food. A baby who has had the correct natural foods introduced at the correct age will grow up less fussy and problematic with meals, and will be healthier and mentally alert.

Avoid chemical, sweetened and artificial juices. Filtered water (as nature intended) and herbal teas are suitable. Occasionally, fresh organic vegetable juices, and **very occasionally**, diluted freshly squeezed organic fruit juices may be given.

CLOTHING

Clothing is another issue which could create discomfort, causing the child to cry, leading to misunderstood 'language'. The baby has been growing in the womb for many months with ample space for movement, until that space became limited due to growth. Once born, babies sleep continually and take comfort from being wrapped up tightly, as it gives them the security they enjoyed in the womb. When awake, their new-found freedom calls for exploration, and they should be given the opportunity to stretch, as this is a form of exercise needed to strengthen their muscles and get their lymphatic fluids and blood circulating. As they grow, they should be allowed more and more freedom, as babies weighed down with excessive and restrictive clothing, will find it difficult to move and exercise.

HOLDING BABIES

Many family and friends visit to view and enjoy the newborn. Normally baby is passed around from person to person. Each person has an entirely different hold or grip on the baby. Very often this can cause discomfort to the new-born, which is displayed by restlessness and crying - frequently in the evenings at bedtime. Many people will understand if explained why baby's 'passing around' is limited to only a few selected persons.

PLASTIC BABY BOTTLES

Bisphenol A (BPA) is a chemical agent used in manufacturing many baby bottles. Heated temperatures cause Bisphenol A to leach into the fatty particles of milk contained in these bottles. Acid drinks such as apple juice also cause it to leach into the liquid content. Bisphenol A mimics estrogen and it is believed by some that long-term and excessive exposure may cause hormonal imbalances in the human body, especially during growth stages (as with babies and children). Make certain that EVERYTHING (plates, cups, toys) used by children is BPA free, which is difficult to confirm as it is not stated on items. Phone manufacturers and obtain confirmation.

CHAPTER 5
TODDLERS, PRESCHOOLERS AND ELEMENTARY SCHOOL CHILDREN

TODDLERS AND PRESCHOOLERS

FUSSY TODDLERS AND CHILDREN

I cannot begin to mention how many times I have been contacted by concerned mothers, whose children are fussy and will not eat. My concern is not that children are fussy, but that they have been fed junk and convenience food, and when it is finally meal time, mothers expect children to "sit down and eat your food!" Another major concern is the quality of food supplied to children that lack the nutrients required to strengthen and nourish their immune system. When I see what children eat, I am aware that those foods will lower their resistance, resulting in low-grade illnesses, and as they grow, their weaknesses will develop with them.

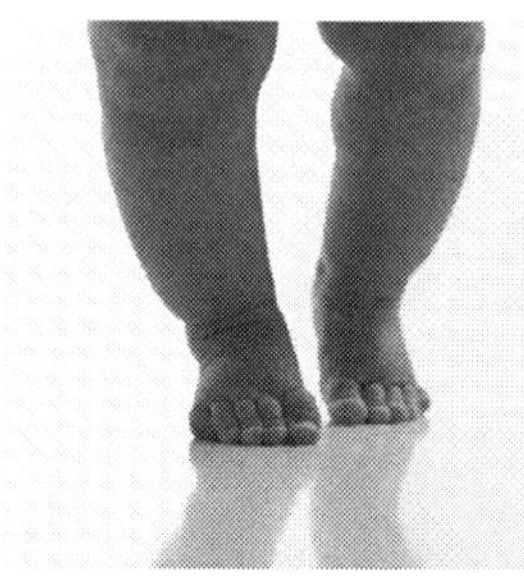

Mothers tell me that they cannot get their children to eat 'good' food. I tell them that babies and small children do not do the grocery shopping, nor do they prepare the foods. They mere eat what's given to them. Fussy children are created – not born that way. For this reason, it is so important to introduce them to foods as described in the previous chapter.

Fortunately, there are ways to correct these situations. Do not be concerned about fussy toddlers who seem unwilling to eat, as no child will starve willingly. Do not make a fuss about meals or allow food to become an issue. As the child is playing, cut small amounts of food (e.g., half a banana sliced, quarter of an apple cut into pieces, a few raisins), and places it next to where the child is playing. Announce that it is there to be eaten, and casually add that it may be shared with the toys. Walk away and leave the child.

When no fuss is made, the child will eat, even if only one piece of substance is consumed. Gradually this will increase.

Do not bribe or reward children with candy, cookies, carbonated drinks and other undesirable foods. This could lead to permanent bad eating habits, which will have a detrimental affect on their immune system.

Chemical and refined foods containing artificial colorings, preservatives, flavorings with refined sugar contribute greatly to hyperactivity, lack of concentration, behavioral problems, aggression, lack of coordination and many other performance disorders. Excessive salt and sugar must be avoided. Fresh and dried fruit, root vegetables and raw honey are healthy sweet foods and sweeteners.

Because of their rapid growth rate, toddlers need more protein than adults. Due to the adverse affects of growth hormones, steroids and antibiotics, only organic protein should be fed to children. Animal fats should be reduced, but natural fats (nuts, seeds, avocado, olives, and coconut) should be supplied. If children with no dairy intolerance are given cows milk, they should have organic full cream milk, and not skimmed milk.

ELEMENTARY SCHOOL CHILDREN

The foundation of the child's future health and eating habits is laid at baby and toddler age, hence an introduction to natural foods at this crucial age is of the utmost importance. It is impossible to keep a child away from 'treats', and care must be taken that they are not made outcasts or labeled as 'different' by their peers, and even their friend's mothers who may not want to prepare special meals for the child when they are invited to play. To prevent this, an easy guideline may be to allow the child to eat a little of what the friends eat when they are out to play, but control their eating habits at home. Control it further by having their friends over to play, rather than them out to play. Children well-rounded in natural foods will often personally choose not to eat their friend's food, and refuse what they are offered. When their friends come to visit, continue to serve the foods the family is accustomed to, and do not break the rules for the friend's sake, as good habits are easily broken and difficult to restore.

SUSTAINED HEALTHY LIFESTYLE: There are many ways to approach healthy nutritional lifestyles with children, and it is advisable to select the options suitable to the family. Herewith are merely two options:

1) Remain ridged with healthy nutrition and don't compromise under any circumstances. Feed the family only organic foods, disallowing 'junk' at all times.

2) Compromise **slightly** for various reasons.

One reason could be to introduce children to reality of what is in the world, educating them to make healthy choices, thus preparing them for later years. This will give them an introduction to both worlds (healthy and junk food). Guide them back to correct choices if the situation gets slightly out of hand.

Another reason could be to prevent them from being labeled'different' or 'weird' by other children or society.

A general rule that works well to compromise **slightly**, is if children know they have to eat their 'healthy' food during the week (and no other compromises are made) but are allowed a few exceptions over the weekend. The exceptions need not necessarily be junk food to the standards or the normal 'junk world'. There are pure chocolates, organic ice cream, healthy hamburgers and pizzas (even homemade), pure fruit or vegetable juices, that may be allowed in moderation, over the weekend.

BIRTHDAY PARTIES: These are always a problem for health conscious families. These are two suggestions to address the situation:

1) If in fear of labeling children by sending them to a birthday party with rice cakes and raisins, avoid them eating too much junk at the party by feeding them a nutritious meal before they leave. They will then only 'pick' at the food

without it being obvious that they are not allowed to eat the junk. This works very well for children who are more sensitive and shy.

2) Another approach is to explain to the hostess that the child is allergic or sensitive to wheat and chemicals, and to avoid a reaction they have to abstain from food containing these. Then packed foods such as carob and nut bars, dates, nut and raisin clusters with a pure fruit juice are appropriate. The other children at the party would probably want to try these new treats as well.

WHEAT AND WHEAT PRODUCTS: Wheat is a major contributor to allergies and food sensitivities which include behavior, stuffy or runny noses, coughs, skin rashes or itches, lowered levels of concentration, uncoordination, hyperactivity, restlessness, asthma, sinusitis, eczema and psoriasis.

Eliminating wheat from a child's diet is easier said than done, as it is difficult sending children to school with salads, fruit and other nutritional foods as these can be messy and lose their freshness. If the children have grown up with these foods as a nutritional habit, then it will not pose a problem, but it certainly is a major issue if a sudden change has to be made.

An easier way of overcoming it is to substitute their wheat sandwiches with whole rye (or other whole grain) bread sandwiches. Alternatively, allow them to eat organic whole wheat sandwiches at school only, ensuring that they do not eat wheat products or wheat based cereals for breakfast, sandwiches again after school when they get home, and further wheat dishes, such as pasta or pizza, for dinner. Their systems will cope much better if exposed to wheat once a day rather than a continual bombardment throughout the day, and allergy or sensitivity responses, will be minimized. Adopt a 4-day grain rotation for maximum effect, not allowing the same grain within a four-day period.

From an early age, get children accustomed to home-made dishes such as soups, vegetable casseroles, stir-fries, salads and fruit salads as well as nuts, seeds, herbal teas and water. This will ensure a strong immune system, allowing them to enjoy health with minimal medical bills throughout their lives.

CLOTHING CHILDREN

It is common practice within a family or circle of friends to hand down items of clothing. When it comes to shoes, some issues to consider are:

- ❑ Shoes are molded according to the shape of the original feet that occupied them. No two pairs of feet are the same, and so the new feet could be influenced by the mold and grow according to the shape of the shoe.
- ❑ Only quality shoes, such as soft leather, should be worn.
- ❑ Purchase for comfort not fashion, or cuteness!
- ❑ Do not allow children to wear shoes they have out-grown to justify the money spent on that item. 'Crippled' feet cost a considerable amount to correct and often the damage is permanent.

In certain parts of the Southern hemisphere, temperatures during the day may drop from 3.00 pm (15.00 hrs) onwards. To prevent children from suffering with upper respiratory complaints, it is advisable to clothe them according to the temperature of the day (and night). Although it is advisable to allow children 'dress freedom', it is equally as advisable to ensure that they are wearing shoes and a sweat suit (or similar clothing) when the temperature starts to decline. This is especially important if the floor of the home is tiled or cold. Use common sense to assess the weather and determine if the child is adequately dressed.

Well fed and well clothed children are happy, healthy children.

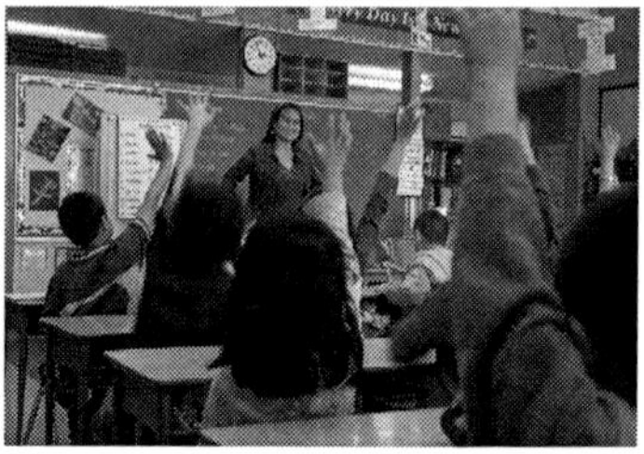

DIET # 2: WHEAT AND SUGAR CONTROLLED DIET FOR CHILDREN WITH ALLERGIES

Allergies and food sensitivities such as asthma, eczema, bronchitis, sinusitis, hay fever; candidiasis; learning or concentration difficulties; hyperactivity; aggressive behavior; runny or congested noses; glue ears; sore throat or stomach.

It is extremely difficult to switch children to a healthy lifestyle from the diet they are accustomed to, and convince them that they are no longer allowed to eat their 'normal' food. This transition has to be done gradually and with wisdom. Firstly, it is necessary to explain to the children that the foods they have been eating have contributed to the condition they have, and that they need to cooperate in order to correct their imbalances. Make them aware that their body needs natural foods to make the healing process effective, and that they will be required to eliminate a large amount of their normal 'junk' food from their diet. Further explain that they will reap the benefit for their efforts, and be able to feel the changes for themselves as their symptoms improve.

I have been advising on nutrition for over two decades, and have found that if the diet advised is too strict, mothers find it too difficult to cater for the children and do not follow it, and then nothing is achieved. The first reaction from the mother is the comment "there is nothing left for me to give my child to eat". Most children who have been living on a diet high in refined foods and sugars have to be educated into the new way of eating, and so a gradual transition is often more effective and lasting than a drastic change. For this reason I have allowed a few *'not permitted'* foods (such as organic wholegrain cold cereals, 100% pure organic peanut butter, yeast spreads, unflavored chips and French fries) for the sake of convenience and wider variety. Often these are the foods, which make the difference between people being able to continue, or not. Children who have eaten sweet, colored, flavored cereals their entire life, find it very difficult to give up their junk cold cereals and eat whole grain hot cereals. I have found that, if allowed 'the lesser of the evils' and they can have organic wholegrain cereal, they are more willing to continue with the new diet, which should become a lifestyle.

Children are continually 'rewarded' or given special treats of candy, ice creams, cookies and other junk and chemical foods and consequently have developed a sweet tooth. Rather satisfy their cravings with fruit - nutritionally that is the best food that can be given to them. It is impossible to take candy away from children completely, but limit their intake and keep them away from colored and chemical candy, ice creams, popsicles, refined cookies and flavored chips, soda pop, cheese curls and puffs. The range is too numerous to list. The rule of compromising **slightly** and allowing 'good junk' food occasionally (like weekends) work well with children. Obviously, the more you control it, the healthier the child will be. It is the law of the harvest: as you sow, so you reap.

FOODS TO AVOID

- ❑ SUGAR and foods containing sugar - jam, canned fruits, canned foods, cereals, canned or bottled drinks, candy, cookies, cakes, pop, chocolates, fruit leathers, popsicles.
- ❑ REFINED FOODS (also called 'simple' carbohydrates) - white rice, pasta, flour, and all products made with flour - cookies, cakes, bread, bread rolls, pies, pizza.
- ❑ COLORINGS, ADDITIVES, FLAVORINGS, PRESERVATIVES. These artificial chemicals interfere with the body's natural chemicals (hormonal or endocrine systems) resulting in mood swings, anger, behavioral problems, depression and even aggression.

PERMITTED FOODS

- ❑ COMPLEX CARBOHYDRATES - organic whole grains, legumes, vegetables and fruit.
- ❑ SUGAR to sweeten herbal teas and hot cereals (porridges): raw honey or raw brown sugar in moderation, stevia.

A good, general rule to remember is: when taking away one food, try to offer a healthy alternative! The following is merely a guideline. Daily food intake should be higher in fruit, vegetables and salads than other foods: 70-80% alkaline and 20-30% acid (refer to Acid/Alkaline Diet #3 for suggestions on breakfast, lunch, dinner and snacks).

NOT PERMITTED	PERMITTED
Margarine and butter spreads	Butter - organic, unsalted in moderation
Cold cereals containing wheat, sugar, colorings and flavorings.	Oatmeal, oat bran, maize meal (grits), sorghum porridge, granola/muesli. Organic wholegrain cold cereal as an occasional compromise.
Cookies, crackers (sweet and salty) and snack products made from wheat.	Oat cookies (refer to recipes), rye crackers and rice cakes.
Bread, bread rolls, bread sticks, cakes, rusks, scones, biscuits, wheat crunchies and other wheat products.	Cornbread, oat and cheese scones, rice flour crunchies, granola/muesli bars.(refer to recipes)
Muffins, doughnuts, pies, pizza, bagels, pastries.	Oat muffins and oat based pizza (refer recipes).
White rice, white sugar, 'sticky' brown sugar.	Brown and wild rice, raw unfiltered honey, raw brown sugar, stevia.
Instant desserts, commercial custard and gelatin desserts	Tapioca or sago dessert, home-made custard.

NOT PERMITTED	PERMITTED
Flavored ice cream or yogurt with chemicals. Popsicles (contains sugar, chemicals and colorings)	Organic or home-made ice cream (refer to recipes), live cultured plain yogurt with fresh fruit, honey and nuts (optional). Home-made popsicles (100% pure fruit juice frozen in small containers
Ordinary tea and coffee. Colored and flavored drinks made with hot or cold milk, or water.	Herbal teas. Herbal coffee substitutes - in moderation.
Milkshakes, hot chocolate, artificial 'shakes' and drinks	Fresh smoothies. Organic whole milk - if no allergies.
Dairy based orange juices, cordials and artificial drinks mixed with water. Frozen or canned juices. Regular or diet carbonated drinks.	Filtered water. 100% pure fruit juices (dilute with water).
Processed foods, lunch meats and processed cheese. Chicken, meat, fish, eggs and dairy products that contain hormones, antibiotics, chemicals and colorings.	Organic chicken (cage free), fish (wild) and red meat (grass fed). Eggs (cage free and organic). Tuna, salmon and other seafood (deep water). Cottage, feta, goat's milk and uncolored cheese (natural; organic, hormone and antibiotic free).

NOT PERMITTED	PERMITTED
Flavored chips. Flavored (microwave) popcorn. Flavored cheese curls and puffs.	Unflavored popcorn. Use dry-popper; sprinkle with olive oil and herbal salt. Unflavored, lightly salted chips (in moderation).
Soy products and other fast, convenience foods.	Fresh vegetables, salads and fruit.
Dried fruit with preservatives pickles and mushrooms. Peanut butter that is not 100% natural. Jam, chocolate spreads and other sandwich spreads.	Fresh fruit. Sun-dried fruit. Nuts: almond, hazel, pecan, Brazil, cashew, macadamia. 100% Natural peanut butter, almond or cashew spread; Tahini (sesame seed paste). Raw honey in place of jam.
Beef stock spreads. Shakes with chemical ingredients, sugar and colorings.	Yeast and vegetable spreads. Nutritional shakes **without colorings, preservatives, soy and refined sugar.**
Commercial mayonnaise. Commercial salad dressings. Commercial sauces, pickles, chutney.	Home-made mayonnaise, vegetable grapeseed (vegan) mayonnaise (health food store). Home-made salad dressing, home-made sauces (use corn starch to thicken).

SCHOOL LUNCHES

Several of these points have been mentioned previously, but because they are *that* important, they need reiterating.

The biggest problem I have encountered with mothers catering for children with wheat sensitivities and allergies are packed school lunches. When a mother is instructed to eliminate wheat from the child's diet she is faced with an enormous problem, as it is difficult to switch a child over night from sandwiches to salad. Most often the child 'cheats' at school anyway and eats a friend's sandwiches. I have found that the following approach works in most cases, and recommend parents try it. Give the child sandwiches for school but avoid wheat products (toast, rolls, buns, wheat porridges or hot cereals) at breakfast. Rather give the child oatmeal, maize meal (grits), granola/muesli, fruit and yogurt, or anything else that is nutritious and wheat free. When the child returns home from school, give them lunch such as an omelet, corn on the cob, oat based pizza, soup or anything else that is nutritious and wheat free and avoid giving sandwiches, bread or any other wheat products. The evening meal can again be wheatless with foods such as brown rice, sir fries, stews, protein and vegetables.

Many mothers have achieved the desired results by limiting the child's wheat intake to once a day only with sandwiches at school. It is very important that the child avoids wheat over weekends, and as much as possible, during school holidays. Remember that the more wheat is avoided, the better the results. If a child is gluten sensitive, then wheat, oats, rye and barley must be avoided as well.

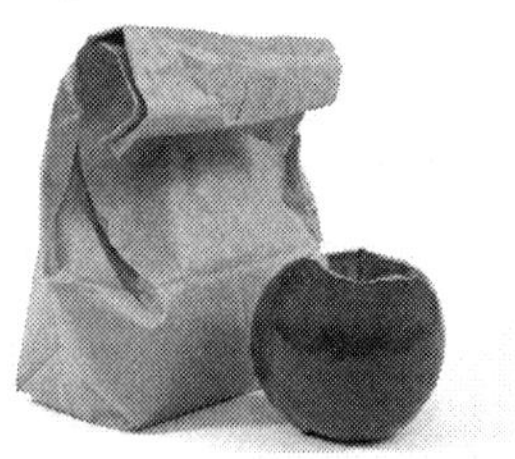

At this age, children are not able to help themselves. As parents, we ***have to*** do the best we can to give them the best health possible. It does take patience, creativity, convincing, bribing, pleading, and most of all – love!

CHAPTER 6
ADOLESCENTS

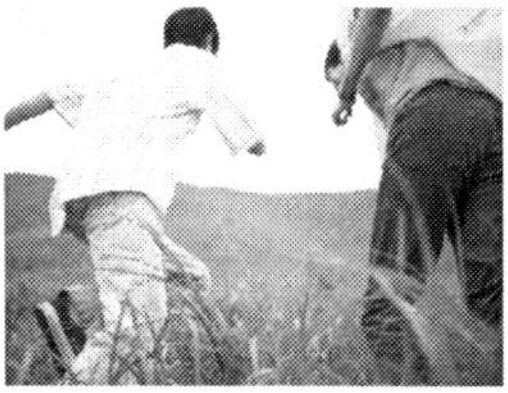

At this age, children are dealing with rapid growth spurts and therefore need more protein - emphasizing plant protein and limiting animal protein. Boys need more protein than girls do. Boys seem to develop 'holes in their stomachs and hollow legs' as they snack continually, devouring whatever they see. Teenagers are seldom present for regular meals and prefer to snack while 'on the run'. It is extremely important that the home has readily available home-made meals, fruit desserts (smoothies), attractive vegetable dishes, snacks and healthy treats, as they will eat what is available.

If the home is stocked with candy, cookies, chips, ice cream, and other foods which are low in valuable nutrients, vitamins and minerals but high in sugar, salt, fat, preservatives and other additives, children will eat these foods and the foundation for future diseases will be laid. These include heart diseases, osteoporosis and other arthritic disorders, colonic and digestive imbalances. Acne eruption will be prevalent.

Alexander Schuss, an American criminologist, researched and wrote the book *"Diet, Crime and Delinquency",* showing that additives, junk food, refined sugar and carbohydrates lead to delinquency and bad behavior in juveniles. Apart from his work, many case studies show that refined sugar and carbohydrates can lead to aggression, lack of concentration, hyperactivity, lack of coordination and learning problems.

Many teenagers are at a vulnerable age and may change their dietary habits and become vegetarian, or adopt the more drastic measures of anorexia and bulimia. The latter two would be avoided if the children have grown up eating healthy food, and will then have no reason to resort to starvation or vomiting to reduce overweight caused by refined and junk food.

Adolescents, who have no skin problems, are advised to follow the Acid/Alkaline Diet (# 3).

ACNE

Acne vulgaris is a common skin condition that probably causes adolescents the most stress, and destroys confidence more than any other factor. Textbooks teach that this condition is caused by over active hormones and sebaceous gland secretions.

Acne lesions can be either inflamed or not, and can cover areas from shoulders, neck, face to forehead. Although mostly common with adolescence, it can continue till any age, or return as geriatric acne at a mature age.

Many factors are credited as the cause of this skin condition ranging from genetic disorders, hyperactive hormones and sebaceous glands, to stress and the use of different drugs. According to my observations, as well as dealings with sever acne cases, refined carbohydrates are the main culprits. Many teenagers practically survive on these high sugar foods, which over stimulate insulin production due to excess blood sugar. The resulting high levels of testosterone (for both male and female) secreted from the adrenal cortex, activates sebum and keratin production. Excessive sebum and enlarged pores lead to open blackheads and closed whiteheads. These comedones become enlarged and sometimes inflamed due to bacteria from the pus of dead white cells.

THE 'EXCESSIVE' FACTORS

Simply stated, the acne pattern is laid out as follows: excessive carbohydrate intake leads to high blood sugar. Excessive blood sugar (hyperglycemia) causes the excessive secretion of insulin from the pancreas. Excessive insulin levels in the blood trigger excessive testosterone secretions (androgens) from the adrenal cortex, which in turn, triggers excessive secretion of sebum from sebaceous glands. Excessive sebum blocks skin pores which develops into acne lesions that may (or may not) become inflamed.

I have witnessed many, as well as severe, cases of acne clear up completely with a change in lifestyle that requires the following three rules:

Rule 1) Avoid all forms of refined carbohydrates (*no matter what temptations* are experienced). This is *the* most important rule.

Rule 2) Eat natural foods *at all times* such as vegetables, salads, fruit, sprouts, nuts, seeds, organic whole grains and legumes; Organic animal protein and dairy products. Drink only water and herbal teas.

Rule 3) ***Avoid all forms of refined carbohydrates……***

CONCLUSION:

Acne sufferers who cut out refined carbohydrates (candy, sodas, cookies, bread, pasta, crackers, chips) will not only clear up their condition, but will also enjoy the benefits of losing excess weight. Both these factors lead to a happier existence.

CASE STUDY:

Male, aged 18 came to consult with me regarding his severe acne. This was undoubtedly the worst case I had ever dealt with. Due to his condition, he had never had a girlfriend and was socially withdrawn. After explaining the logistics of acne to him, he committed to follow the diet.

One month later his skin cleared approximately 60%. After another month, his skin was clear, and he showed a few scars evidencing the disorder. I formulated essential oils to treat those.

Three months after his first consultation, he was dating his first girlfriend. Within a couple of months, he was engaged.

He admitted that the change in lifestyle was not easy but he had to make a choice – eat as he normally does and live with his condition, or make an effort to correct it. Fortunately, he made the right decision.

CHAPTER 7
ADULTS

The body needs to receive a balanced diet to enjoy good health. Too much or too little of either acid or alkaline can cause imbalances such as food allergies, respiratory complaints and anemia, to mention only a few. To maintain a normal healthy balance, the **Acid/Alkaline Diet (#3)** is recommended with a 70-80% intake of alkaline foods and a 20-30% intake of acid foods. Acid foods are necessary, but there is a vast difference between **'good acids'** and **'bad acids'**. **Good acids** are plant proteins (organic whole grains and legumes); certain nuts and fruits; organic, hormone free dairy products (in moderation) and organic, hormone free animal protein (for those who are not vegetarian). **Bad acids** are tea, coffee, sugar, bread, pasta, cakes, cookies, candy, chocolates, soda and the host of 'dead' foods made with refined ingredients, sugar and artificial ingredients.

The following explains the concept of acid/ alkaline.

ACID / ALKALINE

We measure liquids to establish their degree of acidity or alkalinity by using litmus paper. Blue litmus paper turns red in the presence of acid, and red litmus paper turn blue in the presence of an alkaline solution. A number and the letters **pH** express the resulting degree of acidity/alkalinity. pH relates to the number of positively charged hydrogen ions present in any liquid solution. 'p' stands for potential and 'H' for hydrogen. The numbers range from 0 to 14. Anything below 7 indicates the degree of acidity, 7 indicates neutral, and anything above 7 shows the degree of alkalinity. Thus, a fluid which is around pH 3.5 would be very acidic, while something with a pH of 6.5 would be barely acidic. Blood should have a pH balance of 7.4, making it slightly alkaline.

ACID BUFFER

Foods are classified as being either alkaline or acid. If our diets are high in refined foods, coffee, tea, sugar, carbonated drinks and other processed foods, we become acidic. The process of homeostasis does what it can to restore the pH balance to normal; otherwise our bodies would become too acidic, leading to acidosis, disease and ultimately death. If we do not provide sufficient alkaline foods in our diet, the body, through the process of homeostasis, extracts calcium (which is an alkaline mineral) from the bones (where calcium is stored) to restore blood to its required alkaline balance. This continual process of calcium depletion eventually leads or contributes to osteoporosis.

ALKALINE BUFFER

If the body became too alkaline, the heart would go into spasms, leading to death. As most natural foods contain potassium, nature has provided a way for us to lose the excess potassium through the adrenal cortex, which secretes aldosterone. This hormone controls our sodium and potassium levels by allowing the body to lose potassium and retain sodium. For this reason, it is a heath hazard to add extra salt to foods as it will affect our blood pressure.

In perfect health, our body fluids (blood, lymph, saliva) should be slightly alkaline. If they were acidic, severe health problems could result, including coma and even death. Should alkalinity be too strong, tetany and convulsions are likely to occur.

pH LEVELS OF BODY FLUIDS

Blood: arterial - 7.4; venous - 7.3

Saliva - 6.8 to 7.1 (slightly more acid but still alkaline)

Digestive juices - 8.8 (produced by the pancreas)

Gastric acids - 1.5 (found in the stomach and may vary from person to person)

Bile - alkaline

Pancreatic digestive juices - alkaline at 8.8

Intestinal digestive juices - alkaline

Skin - acid at 5.5

Urine - acid to slightly alkaline ranging from 4.5 to 7.5

Signs and symptoms of lowered stomach acidity are noticeable indigestion symptoms directly after eating, such as bloating, heartburn, belching, together with an uncomfortable full feeling, multiple food allergies, rectal itching, nails which flake and crack, anemia and acne.

EXTREMES OF ACIDITY AND ALKALINITY

ACIDOSIS is a condition, which develops in certain disease states such as uncontrolled diabetes, some forms of kidney disease, or after acute diarrhea or vomiting. The effect of a blood pH of less than 7 can be dramatic. Symptoms involving the central nervous system can rapidly manifest themselves, including giddiness, palpitations and breathing difficulties, numbness and tingling, visual disturbances, nausea, extreme fatigue and ultimately loss of consciousness and coma. It is not necessary to have one of these conditions to experience the effect of acidosis.

ALKALOSIS is when there is an excessive accumulation of alkaline in the blood. This condition is far less common, and is often the result of the abuse of bicarbonate of soda or other alkalizing medications used for stomach acidity. Alkalosis ultimately affects the nervous system causing cramps, muscle spasms, tetany and even epileptic seizures. Although alkalosis is less threatening, if the breathing or heart muscles are affected, death can follow. I warn, and am strongly against the oral ingesting of alkaline forming substances such as potassium tablets. Rather maintain balance by eating as nature intended, as natural foods are formulated, by nature to balance us.

To accurately summarize acid/alkaline foods, it is necessary to consider the fact that certain foods classified as acid, are alkaline forming in the body. For example, lemons are classified as acid but have an alkaline tendency. All **fresh** citrus fruits contain citric acid and so they are acid in status but alkaline in potential once they have been metabolized, and are therefore an alkaline forming food. Citrus fruit picked and left in storage or uneaten, lose their energy vibrations as they age and become acid forming.

The process of digestion causes all foods consumed to form water, inorganic compounds and dioxide. Inorganic compounds that have more potassium, calcium and sodium are alkaline forming. Inorganic compounds that have more chloride, sulphur and phosphate are acid forming.

More simply explained, the mineral elements in food contribute towards the acid/alkaline status and the following basic minerals are examples:

Minerals most commonly found in alkaline foods: sodium (Na), calcium (Ca), potassium (K), magnesium (Mg), iron (Fe).

Minerals most commonly found in acid forming foods: sulphur (S), phosphorus (P), chlorine (CI), iodine (I).

Eating proteins bring about sulphuric and phosphoric acid, and eating carbohydrates or fats produces acetic and lactic acids. These need to be eliminated or neutralized as they are potentially dangerous, and sodium, calcium, magnesium and potassium found in alkaline forming fruit and vegetables have the ability to do this. A diet of foods high in acid forming proteins and carbohydrates and low in alkaline forming fruits and vegetables leads to a rise in acidity as well as to dis-eases and diseases, including cancer and heart disease, due to the deficiency of these alkaline minerals.

According to the macrobiotic diet, if potentially acid forming grain-based foods are chewed well (100-200 chews per mouthful), the salivary amylase (ptyalin) which is alkaline, has the ability to change the acid food to alkaline so it will not lead to acidity. Chewing foods well, and coating fruit and vegetables juices (smoothies) with saliva before swallowing, will assist not only towards the process of digestion, but also towards pH balance.

ACID AND ALKALINE FOODS

Note: Eating only alkaline foods is just as unadvisable as eating vast amounts of acid foods; for this reason it is important to maintain a balance of acid and alkaline foods in the diet.

ACID FOODS

(Foods marked with * are rich in potassium.)

ANIMAL PROTEIN: Red meat, venison, poultry, fish and seafood.

All animal protein, including animal products (i.e. dairy products and eggs) should be organic, hormone, steroid and antibiotic free; grass-fed and grass-finished.

Beef should be grass fed, chicken should be cage free and fish should be wild and from deep ocean waters (not farmed).

FISH: Herring, hake, kingklip, mussels, prawns, salmon, sole, trout, tuna, shrimp, lobster, snail, caviar, plus other fish not listed. Avoid crumbed or pre-prepared frozen fish, meat and other foods.

DAIRY PRODUCTS: Cottage cheese, natural live cultured yogurt, butter, cream, goat cheese, feta, uncolored cheese. Milk (Because cattle are grain fed, given hormones, and milk is pasteurized and homogenized, the molecular structure changes and milk becomes mucus forming.)

GRAINS: Maize meal (grits)*, oatmeal* & oat bran*, barley*, rye*, brown rice, sorghum, granola/muesli.

HERBAL COFFEES SUBSTITUTE: Although a good substitute for coffee, they are still acid forming and should be consumed in moderation.

MISCELLANEOUS: Eggs, mayonnaise (home-made), yeast spreads, olives, pickled onions, gherkins and other pickled products; grape, balsamic, apple cider and other vinegars.

LEGUMES / PULSES: Peas, peanuts, fermented soy beans, fermented tofu and lentils. Most soy beans are genetically modified. Soy *products*, due to processing, are acid (as are all processed foods), and are certainly not recommended as a health food. Genetically engineered soy beans, and products made from these, should be avoided. I personally do not encourage the consumption of soy due to its link to breast cancer (and in my clinical experience) skin rashes and conditions.

NUTS: Brazil, hazel, pecan, walnuts, macadamia, cashew*.

FRUIT: Most fruits should be alkaline, but it depends on what the farmers do with them, e.g., bananas are rich in potassium but often picked green, dipped in a chemical and artificially ripened, so instead of containing potassium, they now contain large amounts of sodium. Most fruits (and vegetables) are irradiated for longer shelf life and placed in cold storage. Fresh fruit straight off the tree is alkaline, except apples which are sprayed continually (I am told approximately 23 times) from a blossom until a fruit and may contain sodium instead of potassium as a result. Chemicals can often be tasted when eating apples.

Acid fruit: Gooseberries, passion fruit/granadilla, grapefruits, guavas, lemons, limes, litchis (lychee), mandarins, oranges, pomegranates, quinces, strawberries, tangerines, kiwi fruit, pineapples, melons, watermelons, sweet melon.

OILS from grains: Cold-pressed wheat germ, corn.

SUGAR: White, brown, molasses, maple syrup, raw honey and agave. (White or 'sticky' (caramel) brown sugar and agave are refined sugars and not recommended for use.)

ALKALINE FOODS

VEGETABLES: Avocado, artichokes, asparagus, eggplant/brinjal, beans, bean sprouts, beetroot, broccoli, cabbages, carrots, cauliflower, celery, zucchini/courgette (baby marrow), cucumber, garlic, green peas, squash, leeks, lettuce, corn, mushrooms, onions, parsnips, parsley, potatoes*, pumpkin, peppers, spinach, sweet potatoes or yams, turnips. Vegetables not listed may also be used, as *all* vegetables are alkaline.

VEGETABLE JUICES: Carrot, cucumber, beetroot, celery.

FRUIT: Most fruits - eat in season.

Sub-acid fruit: apples, apricots, berries, cherries, grapes, litchis, loquats, mangoes, nectarines, peaches, pears, prickly pears, plums.

Sweet fruit: Bananas, dates, figs, papayas, prunes, raisins and sultanas.

HERBALTEAS:*Chamomile, *peppermint,* rosehip,*nettle, *hibiscus,* rooibos, linden flower, comfrey, sage, fennel, honeybush, anise, dandelion, devils claw, parsley. Ensure that teas are herbal and not flavored tea. (Not all herbal teas are listed). Herbal teas have many medicinal values, and remember that fresh is best. Grow herbs in pots or in the garden, and use them in cooking and as teas (optional: sweeten teas slightly with raw honey). You will experience a superior taste of nature at its best.

HERBS AND SPICES: Ginger, garlic, ginseng, thyme, rosemary, fennel. Not all herbs are listed. Use fresh or dried herbs in place of chemical flavorings.

SPROUTS: Germinated beans and seeds are high in nutrients.

NUTS: *Almonds, chestnuts.

SEEDS: Sunflower seeds, sesame seeds, linseed, flaxseed, chia.

GRAINS: millet

OILS cold-pressed from vegetables, seeds and alkaline nuts: avocado, olive, sesame seed, linseed, sunflower, grapeseed, almond.

NEUTRAL SUBSTANCES

WATER: Natural (clean) mineral water has a pH balance of *approximately* 7, but it does vary. The pH of water is affected by geographics, pollutants, mineral and metal content of the water, photosynthesis, acid rain and seasons. Acid rain is when the acid pH of the water is below the accepted natural level which ranges slightly below 5.5 on the pH scale due to nitrogen and sulphur acids. The higher the pH of water, the more environmental friendly it is for aquatic life. The more acidic, the quicker (toxic) metals can dissolve in it. Acid rain and melting snow has a direct affect on the pH balance of lakes and their aquatic life (fish, shrimp and plant life). As the human body is mostly water, it requires natural, clean mineral water with a well balanced pH for optimal functioning. Acid-forming sodas and other chemical compound drinks slowly pollute body systems and cause disease, which may later develop into more serious, painful conditions. Drink water only, as it is what nature intended.

DIET # 3: ACID / ALKALINE DIET

For general daily health, incorporate natural foods.

We are what we eat and we become what we eat. Whatever we eat or drink become our nails, skin, hair, hormonal secretions, etc. There are only 3 things that keep us alive and they are: 1) the air we breathe, 2) the liquids we drink and 3) the foods we eat. We can live without food for a few weeks; without water a few days and without air a few minutes. Nothing else keeps us alive. Nothing else keeps us healthy. Nothing else gives us qualify of life (which is health and energy). We are meant to "eat to live" and not "live to eat". We obtain our energy from the sun. The sun puts energy into plant foods, and by eating natural fresh plant foods such as fruit, salads, vegetables, nuts, seeds, herbs and sprouts, we obtain our energy. People who complain of lethargy, fatigue, pain and ill health are not eating sufficient "nature-made" fresh, natural whole foods, and are eating too many "man-made" (commercially produced) foods that contain chemicals such as preservatives, flavorings, colorings and other chemical additives. These foods are produced with refined carbohydrate such as wheat and sugar, and excess intake cause health problems.

We do not have much control over the air we breathe but we have total control over the liquids we drink and the foods we eat. Only nature-made (natural) foods and liquids are compatible with our body as they are full of essential nutrients such as vitamins, minerals, quality liquids, fibers, carbohydrates, proteins and healthy fats, which are required (and utilized fully) by our body.

Man-made foods are void of quality liquids and fibers, full of chemicals, preservatives, flavorings, additives, refined or chemical sugar, salt, harmful oils or fats, and a host of other damaging agents which are most often destructive to our systems. These ingredients are addictive, cause pain, discomfort, disease, and are often carcinogenic. Natural foods have anti-oxidants, build our systems, prevent pain and disease and give us energy and quality of life. These are all signs of good health. Whatever we eat today is insurance for qualify of life in years to come. We have total control over our health. The choice is ours.

LOW CARBOHYDRATE; LOW ACID AND HIGH ALKALINE DIET

THIS DIET OFFERS RELIEF TO SUFFERERS OF:

Obesity / high cholesterol / poor health in general / low immune system / chronic fatigue / muddle-headedness / confusion / inability to find the right word / unco-ordination / Attention Deficit Disorder (ADD) / hyper activity / poor memory / premenstrual bloating / irritability / depression / premenstrual stress (PMS) / anxiety / headaches / muscle and joint pain / bloating / flatulence / itching or burning in anus / hiatus hernia / indigestion / spastic colon / constipation / diarrhea / irritable bowel syndrome / sexual difficulties / cystitis / fungal infection of nails / athlete's foot / prostatitis / oral or vaginal thrush / lack of libido / vaginitis / skin rashes or itches / skin 'blisters' or peeling skin / psoriasis / urticaria / eczema / acne / lethargy / infertility / low sperm count / bad breath / red, crusty eyelids / ringworm / mood swings / chemical sensitivities / allergies / asthma / insomnia / smelly feet.

Cravings for: sugar, pickles, alcohol, sweet foods, bread or other carbohydrates.

Water blisters on hands, fingers, underneath and side of feet, which itch, pop and peel.

Reaction to: chemicals, fumes, perfumes, or insecticides.

'Movement' or 'gurgling' in the intestines.

ALKALINE / ACID FOODS:

70% of daily consumption (two thirds of food on the plate; or 2 out of three meals per day) should be ALKALINE foods

30% of daily intake (one third of food on the plate; or 1 out of three meals per day) should be good, quality ACID foods

0% of daily intake should be bad ACID foods. To avoid disease, pain, lethargy and ill health, avoid these foods!

GRAINS

Refined grains and sugar are *the* most dis-ease causing food I have come across. For a couple of decades, I have treated dis-eases caused by the excessive consumption of grain products. Twenty years ago, it was mainly wheat to blame; today it is wheat, corn, soy and rice. The reasons are uncomplicated. *The grains eaten are not quality, organic whole grains – they are genetically modified. We eat too many refined grain products – these are all refined, bleached and nutrient depleted. Every meal is loaded with refined grain ingredients.* This bombardment causes an immune response which leads to allergies, skin rashes, eczema, psoriasis, joint pain, indigestion, blemishes, fatigue, and headaches.

To improve on, and avoid these conditions, all grains should be organic whole grain and rotated every 4 days - i.e. do not eat the same grain day after day. Bring in different grains such as amaranth, barley, brown rice, bulgur (cracked wheat), flaxseed, millet, oats, quinoa, rice (brown, wild, basmati, jasmine, black japonica, rye, spelt, couscous, semolina and durum wheat.

Wheat Montana Bronze Chief and Wheat Montana Prairie Gold is the only commercially produced wheat flour I recommend as it is GMO-free, contains no chemicals, nothing added and nothing removed.

SUMMARY: Daily intake of food should consist of:

70% ALKALINE foods	30% good ACID foods	0% bad ACID foods
Vegetables - all **Vegetable juices** (fresh) **Salads** – all **Fruit** – most fruits are alkaline **Sprouts** **Herbs and natural spices** – fresh or dried **Seeds:** sunflower, sesame, pumpkin, chia, flaxseed *. **Seed and vegetable oils** (organic, cold pressed,): olive, avocado, coconut, sunflower, sesame, flaxseed*. **Nuts:** almonds, chestnuts (roasted), coconut (fresh) **Grain:** Millet * Flaxseed is also known as linseed and classified as an 'ancient grain'	**Animal protein** (organic, hormone and anti-biotic free): beef, poultry, veal, seafood, venison, cheese, eggs, dairy. (No processed sausages, deli meats and cheeses.) **Grains:** Corn, oat meal, oat bran, rye, barley, brown and wild rice, sorghum, granola/muesli, **organic** whole wheat **Fruit** – some fruits are classified acid **Legumes or Pulses:** alfalfa, clover, peas, beans, lentils, lupins, mesquite, carob, and peanuts. (Avoid soy, soy products, soy milk and tofu). **Nuts:** pecan, walnuts, cashew, macadamia. **Nut & Legume oils** (cold pressed): Hazelnut, walnut, peanut. (Avoid canola, soy, refined or heat extracted oils).	**Refined carbohydrates:** bread, rolls, bagels, pasta, cakes, cookies, crackers, biscuits, sweets, candy, chocolates, dessert, chips, crisps, microwave flavored popcorn. All foods made with refined ingredients such as flour (of any kind) and sugar. Other foods to avoid: Sausages, honey baked or processed meats and processed cheese. Flavored and artificial dairy products (yoghurt, ice cream). Tea, coffee, soda pop, fruit juices, milk (whole or 2% milk), soy milk. Sugar and artificial sweeteners. Tofu and all soy products. White rice. Alcohol. Refined and heat extracted vegetable, seed and nut oils and fats. Chemical and artificial spices and sauces.

WET AND DRY FOODS

70 - 80% of daily intake should be alkaline, which are 'wet' foods in the form of fruit salads and vegetables. These foods have natural liquids which cleanse the body organs, and in particular, the urinary tract.

20-30% must be **quality** acids which are 'dry' foods in the form of organic protein (preferably plant), grains, legumes and nuts. These foods do contain liquids but many produce oil, which is good if its cold pressed and organic. Grains in particular, should be chewed very well and coated with saliva before swallowing.

Man-made foods are the bad quality 'dry' foods that are harmful to our systems. 'Dry' foods such as bread, pasta, pizza, cookies, crackers, chips, are normally washed down with chemical soda drinks or other (equally as harmful) beverages. To obtain this balance, 70% of food on the plate should be alkaline, and 30% should be 'good' acid; or 2 meals should be alkaline consisting of fruit, salad or vegetables and one meal acid containing grain or protein. It is preferable that meals should always consist of both alkaline and acid. For example, if you have hot cereal (oatmeal) for breakfast, eat fruit at least 20 minutes before your meal; if you eat fish or chicken for lunch, eat vegetables with it; if you eat an organic wholegrain meal (pasta) for dinner, have a large bowl of salad and a small bowl of pasta.

SNACKS

Snack foods should be 'wet' foods and mostly from the 'earth': Fresh fruit, sun-dried fruit, natural yogurt flavored with fruit and nuts, fruit shake, fruit shake and granola/muesli, sunflower seeds and raisins, almonds and other nuts, organic popcorn (dry popper) with olive oil and organic herbs or corn on the cob. As an in-between snack (summer or winter) eat fruit. Alkaline foods should consist mostly of vegetables and fruit. Eat raw foods in the form of salads. Stir-fries or cooked and steamed vegetables should be exposed to heat as little as possible.

The following meal planner is a guideline:

BREAKFAST	LUNCH	DINNER
SUMMER		
1) Fresh fruit salad.	Salad and avocado or corn on the cob.	Grain, protein and vegetables.
2) Fruit, natural yogurt, raw honey, nuts and seeds.	Baked potato or avocado with sliced tomatoes.	Vegetable stir-fry.
3) Granola/muesli and natural yogurt.	Fruit and nuts. Hummus and raw vegetable 'sticks'.	Protein and salad.
WINTER		
1) Oatmeal or maize (grits) porridge (eat fruit first).	Fresh home-made vegetable soup.	Vegetable casserole, pot roast or stew with brown rice.
2) Granola/muesli and yogurt with fresh fruit and nuts.	Baked potato and spinach filling with salad on the side.	Bean soup or cottage pie with fresh vegetables.

Other alkaline products are listed below, giving more examples and what to eat, and what to avoid.

SUMMARY OF ALKALINE AND ACID FOODS	
ALKALINE 70-80%	**ACID 20-30%**
VEGETABLES: all vegetables - cooked or raw. VEGETABLE JUICES: fresh. Preferably juice with pulp	PROTEIN: all animal protein - poultry, meat, fish, seafood, eggs, venison and lamb should be organic and hormone free. Beef: grass fed and grass finished Chicken, turkey, eggs: cage-free Fish - wild or deep sea waters Pork and lamb - pasture raised
GRAINS: millet	GRAINS: organic wheat, rice (brown, basmati, wild), barley, rye, oats, corn, buckwheat, sorghum.
SALADS - with home-made dressings SPROUTS	LEGUMES: organic raw peanuts, peas, beans, lentils, pulses, *organic fermented* soy. Avoid all other forms of soy, soy sauce and soy products
HERBS, HERBAL TEAS & SPICES: fresh is best. Organic dry herbs and spices to flavor foods and enjoy as beverages: ginger, garlic, ginseng, parsley, thyme, rosemary, fennel.	AVOID CHEMICAL SPICES AND FLAVORINGS.

NOT PERMITTED	PERMITTED
FRUIT: most. FRUIT JUICES: fresh. Preferably with pulp	FRUIT: some (refer to acid fruit list). Although certain fruits are classified as acid forming, all fruit become alkaline when digested.
*MILK & DAIRY PRODUCTS: organic, raw goat or raw milk from grass fed cow. Produce from these milks: yoghurt, cheese, butter, cream Home-made almond milk	*MILK &DAIRY PRODUCTS: milk, cheese, butter, yogurt, cream from grain fed cows. MILK: derived from grains and nuts - rice milk, soy milk, cashew milk, store-bought almond milk (due to processing)
SUGAR: Stevia (herbal)	SUGAR in any form: raw brown, raw maple, raw honey and molasses. *Avoid white sugar, agave, syrup, corn syrup and refined honey.*
OILS: cold-pressed from vegetables, seeds and alkaline nuts (sesame, sunflower, linseed, olives and almond).	OILS: cold pressed, unrefined grains oils: corn, wheatgerm.
NUTS: almonds, chestnuts.	NUTS: Brazil, pecan, walnuts, macadamia, cashew, hazel
SEEDS: sunflower, sesame, pumpkin and linseed, chia.	VINEGAR: apple cider vinegar.

*Milk and diary products derived from grain fed cattle that receive hormones and antibiotic, and the milk is pasteurized and homogenized, are acid and mucus forming and contribute to allergies and lactose intolerance.

*Milk and dairy products derived from grass fed cattle that have **not** received hormones and antibiotic, and the milk remains raw, are alkaline forming.

PLANNING DAILY MEALS

SUMMARY:

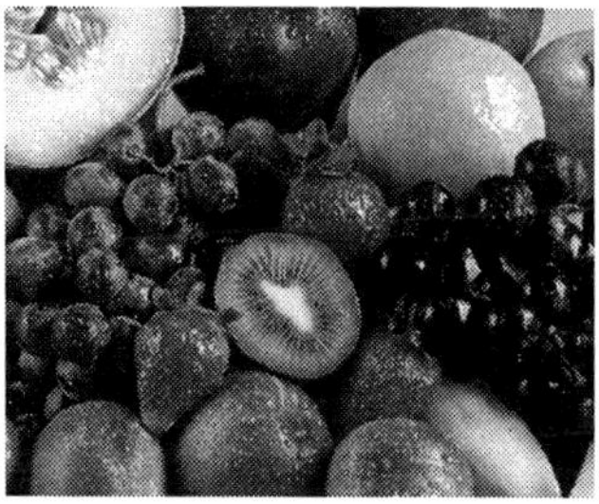

70% Alkaline foods are wet foods in the form of FRUIT, SALADS and VEGETABLES.

30% Acid foods are dry foods in the form of PROTEINS, GRAINS and LEGUMES.

Always eat more plant protein, and keep dairy and animal protein to a minimum as these contain hormones and antibiotics. When consuming animal products, obtain more pure protein such as grass fed beef, cage free chicken and wild (not farmed) deep water fish.

An adequate water intake of 2 glasses during the morning, 2 glasses during the afternoon and a further 2 glasses during the evening, is recommended *especially* when there are dry foods in the diet such as cornbread, oat and cheese scones, rye crackers, rye bread and other whole grain products. If possible, avoid the 'dry' foods mentioned above altogether, as these could lead to constipation if eaten in excess.

From the list below, select foods to plan daily meals. Also refer to the recipe section.

BREAKFAST

Fruit / fruit and unflavored live cultured yogurt / unflavored live cultured yogurt, raw honey and nuts / fruit shake / fruit shake and muesli (granola)/ muesli, yogurt, raw honey and crushed nuts / oatmeal / oat bran / maize meal (grits) / sorghum porridge.

Eggs: Omelet / poached / boiled / scrambled.

Cornbread and raw honey or cream cheese / oat and cheese scones.

A breakfast that will sustain blood sugar, providing energy, vitamins, minerals, carbohydrates, protein and fat is: fresh fruit, unflavored yogurt, raw honey, nuts and seeds (wash nuts and seeds to avoid gas and bloating). (For people who follow food combining, this meal, however good, does not support that).

LUNCH

Baked or boiled potato / potato and mixed green salad / potato and sliced raw tomato.

Salad: greens with raw vegetables / egg / tuna / chicken / brown rice salad.

Avocado / corn on the cob / brown rice and beans.

Left over dinner (sealed in airtight container and refrigerated no longer than 24 hours).

Home-made soup and cornbread: Bean / potato / butternut / carrot / onion / barley / lentils / mixed vegetable soup.

Fruit / fruit and yogurt / fruit shake.

Eggs: omelet / poached / boiled / scrambled (if not eaten at breakfast).

Cornbread and raw honey or cream cheese (if not eaten yet)

DINNER

Vegetables or salad and protein (cage free chicken, wild, deep water fish or grass fed animal protein in moderation) and brown rice.

Casserole / stews / stir-fries / paella / Shepard's pie / rice salad / brown rice and beans.

Home-made soup: Vegetable / butternut / carrot / bean / barley / potato / lentil.

Salad and baked potato / corn on the cob and cornbread.

DESSERT

Fresh fruit salad and plain live culture yogurt or cashew cream, home-made ice cream.

LIQUID

Water mostly. Occasionally: 100% fruit juices (diluted and in moderation), herbal teas (preferably fresh herbs). Herbal coffee substitutes - in moderation as they are acid forming.

ALCOHOL (for those who cannot abstain) Search for slow brewed, low alcohol content beers and wines made with whole ingredients and free from additives, chemicals and preservatives.

SNACKS

Fruit / fruit and unflavored yogurt / unflavored yogurt / fruit shake / fruit shake and (granola) / boiled egg / cornbread and raw honey or cream cheese / oat and cheese scones / baked or boiled potato / brown rice salad / home-made soup and cornbread / corn on the cob / avocado and tomato / sunflower seeds and raisins / almonds or other nuts except peanuts / popcorn / sun dried fruit.

FOOD GROUPS

PROTEINS: Eggs, dairy products, fish, meat, poultry, milk, nuts, seeds, unprocessed cheese, yogurt and soy beans.

PROTEIN STARCH: Beans (blackeye, broad, haricot, kidney, mung and sugar beans) dried peas, chestnuts, peanuts, peanut butter.

STARCH: Barley, bread, wheat, wheat products, pasta, rye, buckwheat, cereals, oats, potatoes, rice, rice cakes, millet, sorghum, tapioca, sago.

MILD STARCH: Beetroot, carrots, cauliflower, corn, squash, artichokes, parsnips, pumpkin, turnips, sweet potatoes or yams.

FAT: Butter, cream, avocado, olives, oil and cold-pressed oils, lecithin spread.

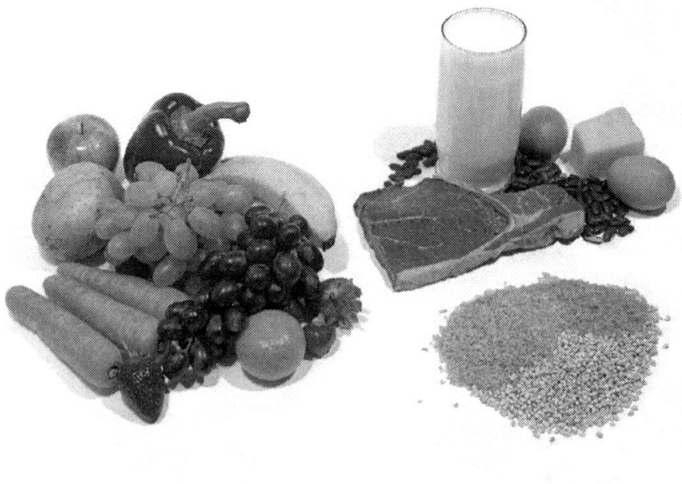

FOOD COMBINING

Food combining plays an important role in health. If desired to follow this lifestyle, the following guideline should be implemented: Eat fruit only with fruit because it digests so easily that any other food will delay digestion and create fermentation. Fruits are classified as:

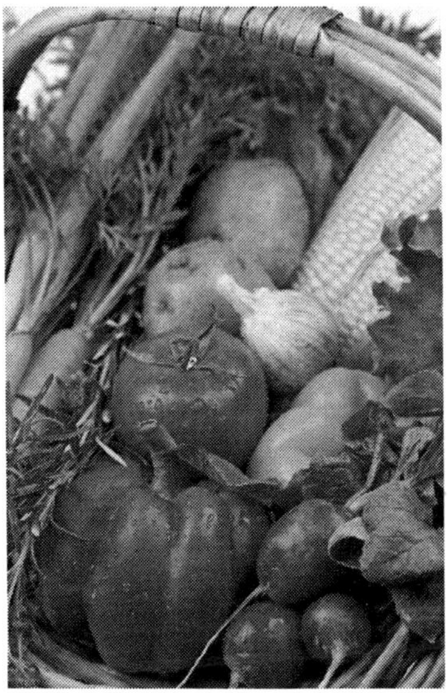

Acid fruit: citrus, pineapple, gooseberry, strawberry, kiwi fruit, pomegranate and quince.

Sub-acid fruit: berries, cherry, grape, passion fruit/granadilla, guava, mango and prickly pear.

Sweet fruit: banana, date, papaya, raisins and fig.

If Stomach sensitivities are experienced, eat fruit from one group only, or from two adjoining groups.

As far as vegetables are concerned, combine starches with each other and some fat can be added in the form of avocado, organic butter or cream, nut butters (almond and cashew nut spreads), cold-pressed oil and olives.

Starches also combine well with green vegetables.

Proteins of various types such as animal and dairy, nuts, seeds or legumes are complex and so different in nature that they should not be combined.

Fat inhibits the digestion of protein and should not be added to protein.

FOOD COMBINING

Acid Fruit, Sub-Acid Fruit, Sweet Fruit

ACID FRUIT ↔ Combine well with sub-acid fruits	***SUB-ACID FRUIT*** Combine well with acid and sweet fruits	↔ ***SWEET FRUIT*** Combine well with sub-acid fruits
Gooseberries	Apple	Banana
Grapefruit	Apricot	Dates
Guava	Berries	Figs
Lemon	Cherries	Mango
Lime	Grapes	Papaya
Mandarin	Litchis	Prunes
Orange	Mango	Raisins
Pomegranate	Nectarine	Sultanas
Passion fruit	Peach	
Quince	Pear	
Strawberries	Plum	
Tangerine	Prickly Pear	
Kiwi Fruit		
Pineapple		
Melon		
Watermelons		
Sweet Melons		

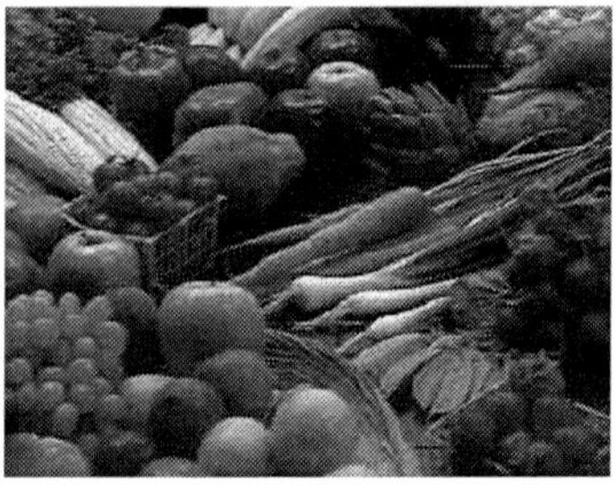

FOOD COMBINING

Protein, Neutral Vegetables, Starch

PROTEIN ↔ Combine well with neutral vegetables	***NEUTRAL VEGETABLES*** Combine well with protein or starch	↔ ***STARCH*** Combines well with neutral vegetables
Beef	Artichoke	Barley
Butter	Asparagus	Bread
Cheese	Avocado	Buckwheat
Coconut	Beetroot	Cereals
Cream	Broccoli	Corn
Eggs	Brussels Sprouts	Millet
Fish	Butternut	Oats
Lamb	Cabbage	Pasta
Milk	Carrots	Potatoes
Nuts	Cauliflower	Rice
Pork	Celery	Rice Cakes
Poultry	Cucumber	Rye
Seeds	Eggplant	Semolina
Veal	Green Beans	Sweet Potatoes
Venison	Lettuce	Wheat
Yogurt	Mushrooms	
	Onions	
	Peas	
	Pumpkin	
	Radishes	
	Spinach	
	Squash	
	Tomato	
	Turnip	
	Watercress	
	Zucchini	

CHAPTER 8
SENIORS

Special nutritional allowances are made for those who have reached a mature age. It is a natural trend as people grow older, they become less active, have less energy and thus food intake decreases. In place of eating a proper meal, especially if living alone, snacks become the meal of the day. Unfortunately there are many constraints due to fixed or low incomes that decrease as inflation increases - forcing many to resort to inexpensive and less quality foods. Possibly because satisfying family is no longer a priority, seniors tend to rely largely on packaged, frozen and other convenience foods.

Hopefully seniors have more time available to prepare meals as home-made soups, casseroles, stews, salads, vegetables and grain foods consist of inexpensive ingredients, and require little preparation time.

Often, to save time and energy, meals are pre-prepare in large quantities and stored in dishes in refrigerators or freezers; not realizing that valuable vitamin C and folic acid are easily depleted through cooking and storing. It is advisable to supplement diets with natural, 'live' vitamins and minerals in order to maintain health.

Problems with teeth could prevent many from chewing nutritious foods like whole grains, fruit with the skin on, nuts and seeds or other fibrous foods. Lack of transport also prevents regular shopping trips. Only for these reasons do I support frozen (or canned) vegetables, fruit and protein rather than resorting to refined and processed foods that store long, but are nutrient depleted and filled with preservatives.

Natural fiber is of particular importance as the elderly are prone to constipation, which in turn leads to other complicated health imbalances. Alkaline foods are also important, as these provide antioxidants that prevent the rapid deterioration caused by acid related ailments such as arthritis, joint and muscle pains as well as the degeneration of the skeletal system. Furthermore, malnutrition will lead to further deterioration of senses such as sight and hearing.

What we eat today will determine our quality of life in years to come; consequently what people ate years ago determined the quality of life they are experiencing today. I basically place senior in three categories:

1) There are many elderly people who enjoy a full life. They are socially active, drive their own vehicles, walk, swim, participate in light sports and share healthy relationships. Independence and quality of life is enjoyed.

2) Others, of the same age, are debilitated and need frequent assistance. Some may use walkers or motorized wheelchairs. Meals are prepared, shopping is done, homes or apartments are serviced and assisted transportation is provided. Some are able to perform crafts, knit, crochet and sew, or participate in board games and watch television. Independence and quality of life is altered according to their health status.

3) Then there are those who are in frail care. Some are bed-bound, others in wheelchairs, and a few on life-support with continuous nursing and medical care. They are fed, bathed and diapered.

Factors that contributed to these variations range from inherited genes, injuries sustained during their lifetime and life-long choices of food. While some abstained from harmful foods, others indulged. Individual choices lead to individual current conditions. Remember, what we eat today is an investment for health conditions we will experience years later – for good or for bad.

GUIDELINES TO HEALTHY EATING FOR SENIORS

- ❑ Eat small, quality snack meals. These will sustain energy and alertness. Small meals are easily and rapidly digested, thus avoiding indigestion.
- ❑ Eat fresh fruit and vegetables. These are alkaline and will reduce the risk of diseases which develop in acid environments, e.g., arthritis.
- ❑ Fruit and vegetables are high in natural fiber and prevent constipation.
- ❑ Drinking adequate quantities (at least 6-8 glasses per day) of filtered water and herbal tea will detoxify the body; prevent constipation and acid-related diseases.
- ❑ Limiting animal protein will lessen the possibility of gall bladder imbalances, heart and other vascular diseases.
- ❑ Avoid bread, cookies, crackers and other refined foods made from wheat. Rather eat rye crackers and rice cakes in moderation.
- ❑ Use cold-pressed olive oil for salads. (Also useful in preventing constipation.)
- ❑ Use organic, cold-pressed coconut oil for cooking.
- ❑ Take a quality multi vitamin and mineral supplement daily.
- ❑ Continue with gentle exercises.
- ❑ Remain interested in hobbies and activities that will stimulate brain function.

CHAPTER 9
CONVALESCENTS

Most people, when they are ill, lose their appetite as the digestive system shuts down' and energy, which would have been used to digest food under normal circumstances, is used to assist in fighting the illness. Once recovered, the convalescent's appetite returns and it is important to nourish the body with nutritious, easily digested substances. Malnutrition is always a risk with prolonged illness and therefore a period of one to two weeks are recommended with the following guidelines:

- Meals should be small in quantity but frequently served.
- Do not combine starch and protein.
- Oatmeal, and other hot wholegrain cereals, for breakfast.
- Fruit, natural yogurt and raw honey as a mid-day snack.
- Vegetable, chicken, barley or lentil soup for lunch.
- Boiled or steamed vegetables, starting with only one vegetable at a time, such as carrots, butternut, peas, sweet potatoes or yams.
- Grains such as barley, lentils or brown rice served with vegetables for dinner.
- Fish - steamed, poached or baked, served as a protein with vegetables in place of grains.
- Skinless chicken or lamb can be added to the diet gradually.
- Nuts, seed and raisins are nutritious snacks (chocolates should be avoided).
- Drink herbal teas or filtered water frequently. Later, diluted pure fruit juices, in moderation, may be added.

Rest and sleep are important, as relaxation is the first stage of normalization, and the body heals itself more rapidly under these conditions.

CHAPTER 10
DETOXIFICATION

DIET # 4: DETOXIFICATION DIET

This detoxification diet is designed to cleanse the body of all undigested and fermented food. Thereafter it is important to watch what is eaten as there will be a rapid build up of toxins again. Headaches and tiredness during the first 3-5 days of detoxification are normal as the body is eliminating waste and it is, in fact, these toxins that are temporarily upsetting the equilibrium. *If necessary* take a pain reliever for the headache, but do not discontinue the diet. Once the headache has subsided, it should not return, and the detoxification period can be completed comfortably.

If you are on medication, **do not** discontinue these. If your medication requires the consumption of food, you will be unable to follow Day 1, which is drinking water only. Simply skip it and commence with Day 2, eating fruit only. If at any time during the 3-day period you feel you are unable to continue with fruit only, proceed to step (3), eating fruit, vegetables and salads. The best benefits are obtained if the diet is followed 100%.

1) **DAY 1**

- ❏ Drink water only. If unable to drink water only, eat fruit (except bananas as they are binding)

2) **DAYS 2 - 4**

- ❏ Any fresh fruit (*except* bananas)

3) **DAYS 5 - 7**

- ❏ Any fresh fruit (*including* bananas)
- ❏ Vegetables – any and all vegetables.
- ❏ Salads and sprouts. (Dressing: freshly squeezed lemon juice and cold pressed olive oil)

4) **DAYS 8 - 10**

- ❑ Any fresh fruit (including bananas)
- ❑ Vegetables - any and all vegetables.
- ❑ Salads and sprouts; Lemon and olive oil dressing.
- ❑ Grains: brown rice, barley, rye, oats, corn.
- ❑ Legumes/pulses: peas, lentils, beans.
- ❑ Nuts and seeds: almonds, sunflower seeds

5) **THEREAFTER**

- ❑ Any fresh fruit (including bananas)
- ❑ Vegetables - any and all vegetables.
- ❑ Salads and sprouts; Lemon and olive oil dressing.
- ❑ Grains: brown rice, barley, rye, oats, corn
- ❑ Legumes/pulses: peas, lentils, beans.
- ❑ Nuts and seeds: almonds, sunflower seeds.

Introduce in *moderation* only if desired:

- ❑ Protein and fat - *organic and hormone-free*: whole milk and cheese, plain live-culture yogurt, butter, cream, cottage or feta cheese. Meat (grass fed) fish (deep ocean water), poultry and eggs (cage-free), venison, pork and lamb (pasture raised).

Liquids:

- ❑ Water - purified or natural spring mineral water.
- ❑ Herbal teas (fresh is best)
- ❑ Herbal coffee substitutes *in moderation*
- ❑ 100% fruit juices - diluted and *in moderation.*

Concentrate more on water and herbal teas. Limit herbal coffees and juices as these are acid forming and not detoxifying.

Avoid: Wheat products: bread, rolls, pasta, pizzas, muffins and cereals. Wheat-based refined foods may cause fermentation to take place in the intestines, as well as constipation resulting in headaches and ill health. If wheat *has* to be part of daily living, have organic whole grain wheat only and keep its intake to a minimum. Practice a 4-day wholegrain rotation, and don't eat wheat until the last of the detoxification steps have been followed.

On completion of the detoxification diet, follow the **Acid/Alkaline Diet (# 3)** concentrating on natural foods only. Avoid manufactured foods.

BENEFITS OF THE DETOXIFICATION DIET

The following improvements will be noticed:

- ❑ Complexion and body skin in general. The skin is an elimination organ, and many toxins are congested in the dermis and subcutaneous layers. As toxins are eliminated, the complexion clears and the skin 'glows'.
- ❑ Weight loss in pounds/kilograms will occur, followed by a reduction in inches/centimeters.
- ❑ Cellulite decreases.
- ❑ Health in general will improve and relief will be experienced from allergy related conditions.
- ❑ Increased energy, with improved concentration and coordination, may be experienced.
- ❑ Reduction in mood swings and emotional outbursts.
- ❑ Halitosis (bad breath) will diminish as the digestive tract rids itself of toxins and fermented food.
- ❑ A general "I feel good" feeling will be experienced.

Case history: Male client aged 40 followed the detoxification diet with such wonderful results that he decided to do it once more. Consequently he lost 24.2 lbs/11 kg, which brought him in line with his desired and normal weight. His health and energy was restored as he continued with the Acid/Alkaline diet.

CHAPTER 11
OBESITY

Any person more than 20% over their normal weight is classified as obese and will be suffering from malnutrition. Any person is at risk of eating themselves into obesity especially with refined and processed foods. Fat babies may become fat children who become fat adults. Obese people have a far greater risk of succumbing to disorders such as high blood pressure, heart disease, circulatory problems, diabetes, atherosclerosis, arthritis of ankles or knees and hips, respiratory ailments, hernias, gall stones, depression and many more conditions.

CAUSES OF OBESITY

- ❑ Bad eating habits.
- ❑ Eating too many 'man-made' carbohydrates.
- ❑ Eating "comfort" foods continually.
- ❑ Eating more calories than can be burned in daily activity.
- ❑ Stress and psychological factors.
- ❑ Childhood obesity resulting from excess consumption 'to please parents'.
- ❑ Nutritional ignorance.
- ❑ Cravings due to allergies.
- ❑ Hormonal imbalances (normally blamed the most but are actually the least cause).
- ❑ 'Kitchen-etic' (not genetic) conditions.
- ❑ Boredom.
- ❑ Nutritional ignorance due to lack of knowledge of what is *really good* and what is *really bad.*
- ❑ Gluttony, self-destruction, lack of concern/self-discipline.

COMBATING OBESITY

The most effective way to lose weight is to:

1. Cut carbohydrates
2. Exercise
3. Adopt an Acid/Alkaline *lifestyle*
4. Count calories

Avoid refined carbohydrates!

STARVATION DIETS

Too often people try to do a quick and drastic weight loss by starving themselves. In nature the body is designed to conserve fat in times of famine. Starvation does not solve a weight problem; it merely upsets the homeostasis of the body, which in turn can lead to health issues such as hypoglycemia. It is far more sensible to make permanent lifestyle changes by following a few simple rules:

1. CUT CARBOHYDRATES

It has already been established that the three food groups we need are carbohydrates, protein and fats and that excess carbohydrates (converted to glucose in the liver) stores in the body's adipose tissue as fat once cells, tissue and systems are saturated with their required energy.

'NO ***BAD*** CARBOHYDRATE' diet should become a life-style and refined carbohydrates and junk food should ALWAYS be avoided. Refined, 'man-made' carbohydrates are foods that increase weight, weaken the immune system and cause dis-ease that lead to either disease or misdiagnosed conditions with unnecessary medications or operations.

For optimal results, I recommend a 'no carbohydrate' diet for at least 3 months but for those who find it impossible, I recommend they start with a 'no carbohydrate' diet for 2 weeks. The more diligent the regiment, the better the results. Ultimately the decision is a personal and individual one.

Once the 'no carbohydrate' diet is completed, then a 70-80% Alkaline and 20-30% Acid forming foods ***lifestyle*** should be followed (refer to CHAPTER 7).

The purpose of avoiding all carbohydrates for 2 weeks (or more) is to "calm" the pancreas and allow hormones in the body to normalize. This reduces cholesterol and glucose levels. The latter will result in weight loss. The reason weight is lost, is because a high carbohydrate diet causes the pancreas to secrete excessive insulin. The body retains water which is needed for the action of hormones. Excessive glucose converts to glycogen (which is heavier than fat) and stores in the liver and muscles. When we reduce carbohydrate foods, insulin secretions normalize and the excess water and glycogen storage is eliminated, causing the body to reduce in weight.

DIET # 5: 14-DAY NO CARBOHYDRATE DIET:

This diet is for optimal improvement in health:

Avoid ALL carbohydrates for 2 weeks (14 days). Carbohydrate foods to avoid include:

- ❑ **Root vegetables:** carrots, potatoes, beets, yams, etc.
- ❑ **ALL fruit** and fruit juices
- ❑ **ALL grains:** oatmeal, corn, wheat, rye, soy, rice, millet.
- ❑ **Refined carbohydrates:** bread, rolls, bagels, pasta, cakes, cookies, crackers, biscuits, sweets, candy, chocolates, dessert, chips, crisps, microwave flavored popcorn. All foods made with refined ingredients such as flour (of any kind) and sugar.
- ❑ **Other foods to avoid:** Sausages, honey baked and smoked meats, processed meats and processed cheese. Flavored and artificial dairy products e.g. yoghurt, ice cream. Tea, coffee, soda pop, fruit juices, soy milk. Sugar and artificial sweeteners. All soy products including tofu. White rice and partially cooked rice/foods. Alcohol.

Refined and heat extracted vegetable, seed and nut oils and fats. Chemical and artificial spices.

The *majority* of daily consumption (70%) should comprise of alkaline foods: salads and vegetables (excluding root vegetables). Included in smaller portions are alkaline nuts, seeds, herbs, sprouts and cold pressed organic oils.

The *minority* of daily consumption (30%) should comprise of only QUALITY acid foods: organic, hormone-free animal proteins and products, legumes/pluses, nuts and cold pressed oils.

70% Alkaline foods:	30% Quality acid foods:
Vegetables - except root vegetables the first 2 weeks. **Vegetable juices** - except root vegetables the first 2 weeks. **Salads** - all raw vegetables except root vegetables the first 2 weeks. **Sprouts** **Herbs and natural spices** – fresh or dried **Seeds:** sunflower, sesame, pumpkin, chia and linseed/flaxseed (an 'ancient grain'). **Seed, vegetable, grain oils** (organic, cold pressed,): olive, avocado, coconut, sunflower, sesame, flaxseed. **Nuts:** almonds, chestnuts (roasted), coconut (fresh)	**Animal protein** (organic, hormone and anti-biotic free): beef, poultry, seafood, veal, venison, cheese, eggs, dairy. (No sausages, processed deli meats and processed cheese.) **Legumes or pulses:** alfalfa, clover, peas, beans, lentils, lupins, mesquite, carob, and peanuts. (Avoid soy, soy products, soy milk and tofu). **Nuts:** pecan, walnuts, cashew, macadamia **Nut & Legume oils** (cold pressed): Hazelnut, walnut, peanut. (Avoid canola, soy, refined or heat extracted oils).

Liquids: Mostly water, fresh vegetable juices (without root vegetables) and herbal teas.

Meal planner example:

Breakfast:	**Snack:**	**Lunch:**	**Snack:**	**Dinner:**
Spanish omelet - or Scrambled eggs with fresh herbs, mushrooms & collard greens.	Cherry tomatoes & cottage cheese	Garden salad with sprouts, avocado & lemon dressing	Celery sticks & almond butter	Chicken & stir-fry vegetables
Boiled egg with tomatoes, cucumber & red bell pepper.	Hummus & raw vegetables	Tuna salad with olive oil &lemon juice (or depending on weather) Vegetable soup	Baby spinach leaves with cucumber and cottage cheese	Baked Fish with steamed or baked vegetables
Plain yogurt, Stevia & nuts	Celery sticks & hummus	Grilled salmon with tomatoes & steamed asparagus	Trail mix made with Almonds, shredded coconut, sunflower & pumpkin seeds	Chef's salad with olive oil and lemon juice (or depending on weather) Fresh vegetable soup.

After 14 days bring back into the diet:

Root vegetables (carrots, potatoes, beets, yams etc.).

ALL fruit (but not fruit juices).

ALL organic whole grains: brown and wild rice, oatmeal, corn, rye, 100% pure rye crackers, GMO free wheat (Wheat Montana Bronze Chief and Prairie Gold). *Avoid soy and soy products!!*

Important: apply a 4-day rotation with all grains (do not eat the same grain without a 4 day break). This will prevent developing allergies.

Continue to avoid: Refined carbohydrates i.e. bread, rolls, bagels, pasta, cakes, cookies, crackers, biscuits, sweets, candy, chocolates, dessert, chips, crisps, microwave flavored popcorn. All foods made with refined ingredients such as flour, soy and sugar.

Other foods to avoid: Sausages, honey baked and smoked meats, processed meats and processed cheese. Flavored and artificial dairy products e.g. yoghurt, ice cream. Tea, coffee, soda pop, fruit juices, soy milk. Sugar and artificial sweeteners. All soy products including tofu. White rice and partially cooked rice/foods. Alcohol. Refined and heat extracted vegetable, seed and nut oils and fats. Chemical and artificial spices.

2. EXERCISE

Good nutrition and gentle exercise is the key to great health! Exercise is especially necessary when any weight loss lifestyle program is introduced. Exercising will tone muscles, sculpt the body and prevent sagging skin. Cardiovascular (aerobics), stretching, resistance training and weight lifting (anaerobic) are all important. Aerobic exercises includes fun activities such as cycling, dancing, jogging, swimming, fast walking, etc. Anaerobic exercises are push-ups, pull-ups, rowing, sit-ups, squats, etc. Individuals need to assess themselves, or have themselves assessed by a professional, and follow their program.

3. ADOPT AN ACID/ALKALINE *LIFESTYLE*

(refer to Chapter 7 for full details)

Diets are short-term, and when the goal is reached, old eating habits rapidly return leading to (an even more) weight gain, unhappiness, depression, health imbalances and loss of confidence. By adopting an Acid/Alkaline *lifestyle* (emphasis on 'lifestyle') which is filled with fruit, salads, vegetables, sprouts, seeds, nuts, organic whole grains, water and other natural foods, will result in good health, more stable emotions and rational thinking, a stronger immune system, good humor, lightheartedness, pain-free living, general wellness together with many other benefits that can be enjoyed.

4. COUNT CALORIES

Once an Acid/Alkaline diet is adopted, it is advisable to count calories. In a very "loose" sense, intake equals output. If we take in more energy than we use, it stands to reason that the excess will be stored. Think of our body as a fuel tank, and our excess fat as a separate reserve tank. If the energy we consume in one day exceeds the energy we expend, we will add fat to our reserve tank and never use our stored energy (fat). To empty our reserve tank, we need to use stored fat by sensibly cutting calories. This can be achieved with the 'no carbohydrate' diet. Thereafter, we need to concentrate on a balanced acid/alkaline diet consisting of natural foods, *not exceeding our daily calorie requirements*. Gentle exercise and good nutrition are the first steps to normalizing and contributing to healthy living. Gentle exercise assists the body's lymphatic, cardiovascular, pulmonary, musculoskeletal and urinary systems whereas strenuous exercises place stress on these systems and their organs. Follow an exercise program at a pace that is suitable, comfortable and achievable.

ENERGY CONSUMPTION ANALOGY

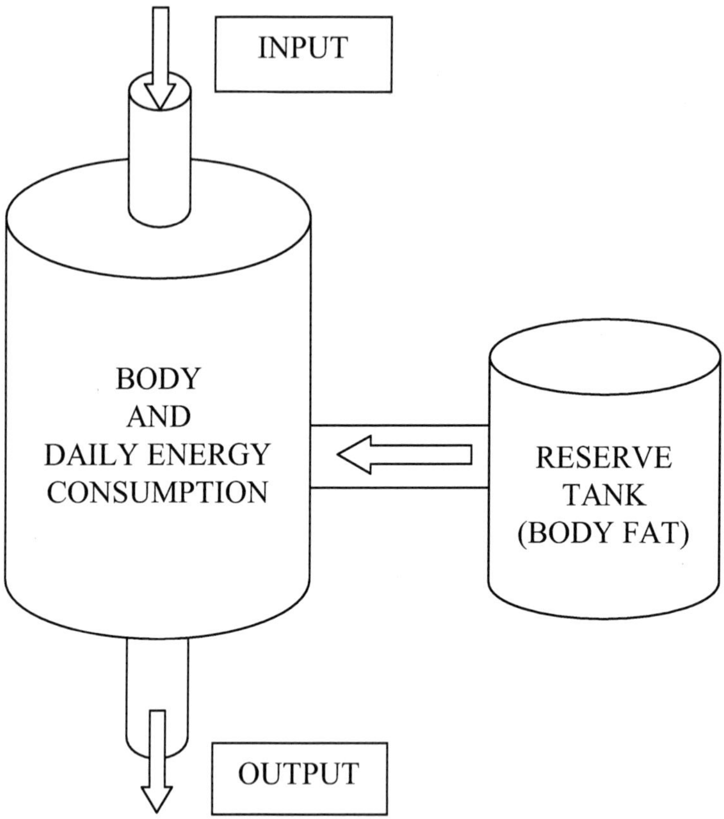

Input equals output - Decrease daily calorie consumption in order for the body to use stored fat.

5. AVOID REFINED CARBOHYDRATES

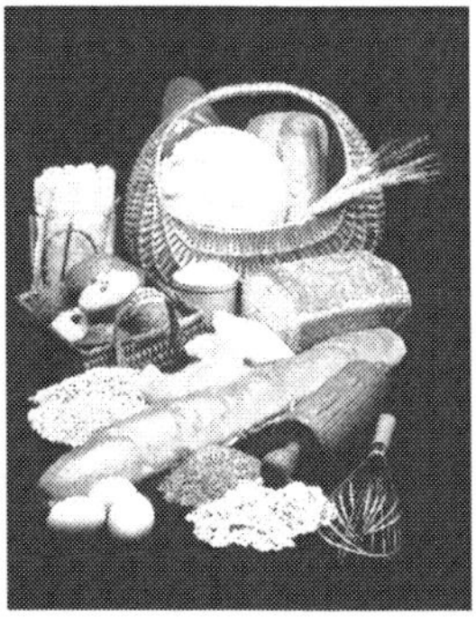

Refined carbohydrates are mostly man-made and it is probably ***the*** single, major cause of imbalances that have afflicted people whom I have, for over twenty years, consulted with. Conditions caused by eating too many refined carbohydrates have presented themselves in the form of fatigue, lethargy, skin rashes or itches, irritable bowel syndrome, depression, constipation, allergies, bloatedness and distended abdomens, muscles and joint pains, mood swings, arthritis, cystitis - just too numerous to list! The conditions are different in many cases, *but the cause remains the same.*

Refined carbohydrates are by and large, manufactured with ingredients that are nutrient depleted, chemically laced, sugar and trans fat saturated. These foods lower the immune system, cause allergy or food sensitivity responses and encourage the uncontrollable colonizing of *candida albicans*.

A lowered immune system attributes to countless conditions that develop within the internal environment of the body. It also directly affects the ability of our systems to protect itself from the external environment, which presents itself in the form of viruses, fungi and bacteria. Allergies and food sensitivities not only cause respiratory ailments, but also cause skin conditions and infections. Candidiasis presents itself in so many aspects that an entire section is devoted to it, within these writings.

I often wonder what it is going to take to make people realize that these delicious tasting foods, that look so attractive and colorful, are directly responsible for many of their health problems that range from the common cold to cancer, with everything else in-between (including weight gain and cellulite!).

CELLULITE

Too often I hear people complain that they are exercising, following a healthy diet, yet they are not losing any weight. Even worse are women who lead an extremely active life, are involved in aerobics, and they have cellulite! The main culprits here are the wrong grains. We are under the impression that all grains are healthy! "Well, they are not!

The more grains we have in our diet (pasta, bread, crackers, chips, white rice) the more cellulite we will have. These foods turn into 'sugar' (glucose) and excess sugar converts to fat. Glucose excites insulin which is a hormone, and hormones play a huge role in the formation of cellulite. When women calm their hormones by adopting a natural lifestyle, cellulite (AND abdominal fat) disappears.

Case History: A woman in her early 30's came to consult with me in my clinic in South Africa. She is a professional aerobics instructor who is slim and beautiful. She exposed her upper thighs and showed me her cellulite exclaiming "Cecilia, I am a professional trainer! I do aerobics 8 hours a day - yet I have all this!!" (grabbing hold of her cellulite).

I asked her to detail her diet and her reply was "I need energy so I carbo-load!" Pasta and "whole-wheat" bread were the major components of her diet together with vegetables and salad. I advised her to go on a 'no man-made carbohydrate' diet and eat vegetables, salads and fruit; and to carbo-load on root vegetables and legumes only. Within 2 weeks her cellulite started reducing. Within a month she had no cellulite!

I can only state that the minute she goes back to her man-made carbohydrate diet, she will get her cellulite back again. I am happy to report that she was more afraid of the cellulite returning than succumbing to her taste buds, so she continued with a natural lifestyle and enjoyed cellulite-free thighs!

SLIMMING DIETS

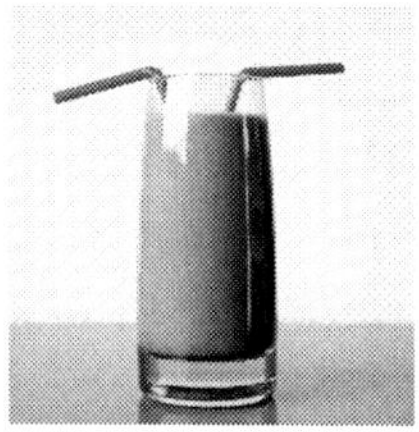

Many slimming diets are drastic and not balanced, and there is the risk of the same weight being gained back due to nutritional ignorance. Slimming diets are designed to make people lose weight but they are not necessarily healthy! They are designed purely for weight-loss and not health-gain. They are acid forming due to man-made ingredients. No drastic measures are needed to shed excess weight. It is the body's natural tendency to heal itself once treated kindly. Any person who changes to a balanced alkaline/acid lifestyle, remaining on whole and natural foods, will not only shed excess weight, but will also reap the benefits of new-found health and energy.

Natural foods, eaten to satisfy and fulfill its purpose, cannot and will not cause obesity or diseases. Good nutrition and gentle exercise is the key to health.

FATS AND REDUCED FATS

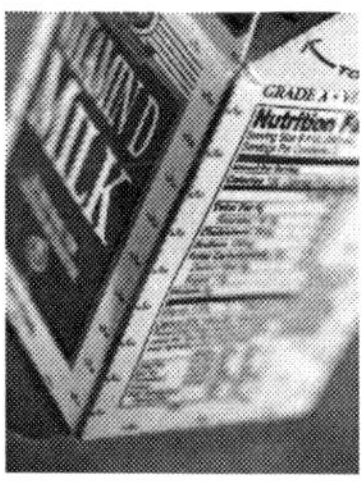

Not all fats are the same and not all fats are bad. Eating the ***right*** fats in ***moderation*** is important. Natural plant fats are very important for *total* health, and *optimal* functioning of body organs and its systems. Too many people focus on the premise that fat is the bad food group that is directly, and singularly responsible for making us fat. Excess MAN-MADE CARBOHYDRATES are the main culprits that make us fat! These foods contain not only bad fats, but refined ingredients as well. Wrong fats (animal fats and hydrogenated oils) make us unhealthy almost quicker than they make us fat. It is more beneficial to eat healthy organic cold pressed natural fats (organic cold pressed olive, coconut, seed and nut oils) in moderation than large quantities of reduced fat products, which are normally laced with chemicals, sugars and refined ingredients as well.

NATURAL GUIDELINE FOR WEIGHT LOSS

Health and weight control is so simple that people do not believe it can exist. To understand the concept, we need to understand creation. We were created by 'nature'. In each religion nature could mean 'someone' or 'something' to that particular person. Nature created the foods we eat, which with ultimate wisdom, are completely compatible with the human digestive system and body functions. All we need to do is learn to eat as nature intended. There are basically three ***natural*** food groups we need to concentrate on:

1. **Carbohydrates** are converted into glucose in the final stage of digestion and used in the body for fuel, energy and heat. Without energy we are depleted and often people complain that they are tired and have no energy. This is due to the fact that they do not consume sufficient energy foods. Natural plant foods obtain their energy from the sun – this is passed on to us when we eat as nature intended.

2. **Proteins** are converted into amino acids in the final stage of digestion and used in the body for growth and repair of bone, muscle, skin, hair and nails. Plant protein is far healthier than animal protein which causes dis-ease and later disease in the human body - especially within the circulatory system. Excess animal protein results in a build up of cholesterol, due to saturated fat which is associated with heart disease, as well as uric acid which causes pain and inflammation in joints.

3. **Fats** are converted into fatty acids and glycerol in the final stage of digestion and used in the body for warmth, protection, energy and the building of cell membranes. Many of our nerve cells have the myelin sheath for protection. Our heart and kidneys are imbedded in a pad of fat for protection as well. Fat is also needed to carry our fat-soluble vitamins A, D, E, and K. *Correct fats are* necessary in our diet, but excessive *incorrect fats* are health threatening. There are 3 groups of fat: **Saturated fats,** found in animal products such as meat, cheese, eggs, milk, butter, cream, dairy and other animal produce. **Unsaturated fats**

(polyunsaturated fats and monounsaturated fats) are from vegetable, plants and fish sources such as olive, grapeseed, wheat germ, sunflower, safflower, corn oil, salmon, and other fish oils. **Trans fats** should be avoided completely as they are hydrogenated or partially hydrogenated, found in many refined foods combined with sugar and chemical ingredients that are not only fattening, but carcinogenic as well.

LIFESTYLE ADVICE

Natural foods were never intended to cause weight gain and ill health. The body is designed to detoxify and heal itself on a continual basis. For optimum health, eat nature-made foods and avoid man-made foods. With the latter, we consume chemicals in the form of flavorings, colorings, additives and preservatives. We do not have digestive enzymes to digest these chemical cocktails and so they accumulate in our systems causing pain, discomfort and disease. Furthermore, these foods contain large amounts of fat, refined oil, sugar, refined flour and other weight gaining ingredients. Our food combinations and *excessive consumption* of these man-made foods cause our weight gain - nothing else.

Any person wanting to enjoy food, health and weight control, must switch their diet to natural foods only. If uncertain which foods are nature-made or man-made, then ask the following question - "was this food that I am about to eat, made by man or nature?" If it grows on a tree, a bush or a vine, if it is from above the ground, under the ground - it is nature-made. On the other hand, if it is in a packet, can, carton or box, off a shelf, or out the cupboard - it is man-made. Man-made foods are dead. They will satisfy taste buds but do very little work within the body systems. They cause allergies, constipation and many other diseases. Nature-made foods build and repair the body, give energy, mental control and clarity. Furthermore, taste buds will come alive and tasting food the way nature intended could be experienced.

Switching to a NATURAL diet will cause weight loss, and improvement with health in general will be noticed. Nature-made foods are all fruits, vegetables (which include salads), grains, nuts, seeds, legumes and herbs. For a detailed list, refer to the **Acid/Alkaline Diet (# 3)**. Drink water, herbal teas and minimize even 100% fruit juices as these are acidic due to processing. To reduce cellulite, avoid ALL wheat products and refined grains.

Athletes who carbo load for energy, must carbo load on potatoes, brown rice, vegetables, beans, corn, barley, legumes and nuts with fruit in between. This will sustain desired blood sugar levels over a prolonged period, and not cause it to plunge the way refined carbohydrates in the form of pasta, bread and white rice, are inclined to do. Follow food combining as described at the end of the Acid/Alkaline Diet.

It is worth mentioning that the more nutrient depleted foods are eaten (such as refined carbohydrates and other junk food), the more hungry a person will get. This in turn, will result in more food (most often junk food again) being consumed. The situation is never ending as the body calls for food, the food supplied is nutrient deficient, the body's needs are not satisfied and once more it will request food through the signals of hunger.

The hypothalamus (situated below the thalamus in the cranial) controls our hunger and satisfaction. Through the actions of the sympathetic nervous system, the hypothalamus will call for food. The excess consumption of these nutrient depleted, refined carbohydrates will cause the liver to convert excess glucose to glycogen - a process know as glycogenesis. Once the glycogen stores (liver and muscle tissue) are saturated, the excess is converted to fat and stored in adipose tissue.

A similar process occurs with excessive consumption of (especially animal) protein. Excess amino acids are deaminated in the liver and the amine group is converted to urea, sent to the kidneys and excreted in the urine while the keto acid portion is used as fuel. or stored as fat.

The converse is true, when sufficient nutrients are consumed, the body is satisfied. There is then no reason for the sympathetic nervous system to trigger any alarms and call for excess food.

The nutrients (vitamins and minerals) contained in fruit, vegetables and other natural foods are sufficient to supply the body with its needs. People, who make this way of eating a life style, eat only to satisfy the need when it is necessary and very seldom snack, or 'look for food'. They are not overweight, have clear complexions and sufficient energy.

GUIDELINES FOR WEIGHT LOSS

- ❑ Eat fruit as a meal or a snack.
- ❑ Avoid saturated fats including animal protein and dairy products.
- ❑ Eat salads often but avoid commercial salad dressings.
- ❑ Drink two liters of water per day (or proportion according to body mass and loss of daily body fluids through urination, perspiration, expiration and fecal elimination).
- ❑ Eliminate all sugar and sugar products.
- ❑ Eliminate refined carbohydrates (bread, pasta, cookies, sodas and juices, pastries, bread, rolls, cold cereals.).
- ❑ Eliminate chemicals (preservatives, flavorings, colorings).
- ❑ Eat vegetables, sprouts, and other nature-made foods.
- ❑ Eat nuts and seeds that are organic and fresh in moderation
- ❑ Implement a gentle exercise program.
- ❑ Burn up more calories per day than consumed. Think of excess weight as a reserve fuel tank. Unless you burn up that excess, you will not lose weight. This can only be done by eating less than the required amount, and exercising more.
- ❑ Do not go on a starvation diet. This will cause the body to believe you are starving, and consequently store weight.

EXERCISING AND ENDURANCE TRAINING

CARBO-LOADING

People who are involved in strenuous activities and endurance sports often 'carbo-load' (i.e. load their bodies with carbohydrates). These 'high energy foods' consist of refined foods such as pasta, white rice and bread. The objective is to store as much glycogen (converted glucose) in muscles as possible, which will later be converted back into a usable form of energy.

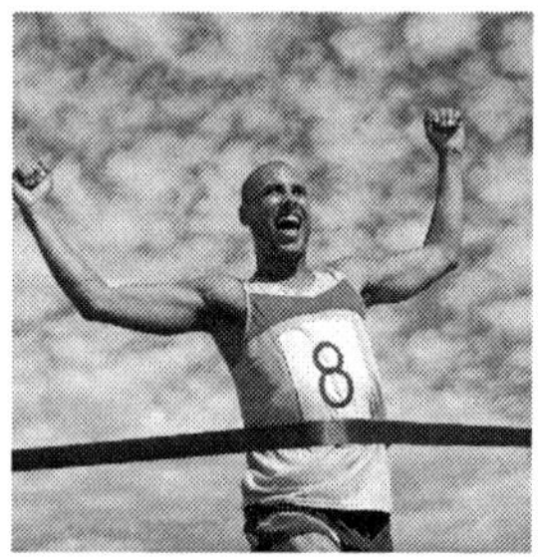

People who wish to carbo-load would do so much better if they loaded with root vegetables (potatoes, yams, carrots, beets) and vegetable proteins such as legumes (beans, lentils, peas, peanuts.). These foods will provide them with sustained energy rather than boost their energy, just to drop it low again as refined foods do.

Case History: A marathon runner in his late 20's, early 30's, consulted with me in my clinic many years ago in South Africa. He was (at that time) a Comrades Marathon runner, which is one of the oldest and most enduring ultra marathon run in South Africa spanning approximately 56 miles (90km). He told me that each year he would almost make the finishing line but he would run out of 'steam', his knees would buckle and he could go no further. He would collapse with exhaustion.

I advised him to immediately adopt a natural diet and cut out man-made foods; drink water and avoid chemical sports drinks. I further advised him to cut out refined carbo-loading and to carbo-load on root vegetables while training, and before the race.

He visited with me at my clinic after the race and told me that not only did he complete the race within an excellent record time, but he felt he could have continued with the race even *after* he reached the finishing line! His change was as night is to day.

PROTEIN DRINKS AND SLIMMING SHAKES

I personally categorize my foods into 'live' and 'dead' foods. As far as I am concerned, powdered protein drinks are 'dead' foods. Many of these drinks are soy based and I certainly would not drink (or eat) any soy product (Refer to SOY under 'FOODS TO AVOID' in Chapter 2). Whey protein is a better selection for those who incorporate protein drinks into their diet. Avoid those with chemical colorings and flavorings.

Slimming shakes are more 'dead' drinks, often laced with artificial colorings and flavorings. When people stop and go back to their normal (bad) eating habits, all the weight is gained back again.

Switch to a natural lifestyle and enjoy all the benefits. Nevertheless, each individual is able to make their own selection with regard to food and beverages. It all comes down to "we are what we eat".

PROTEIN BARS AND 'HEALTH' BARS

I feel the same about protein bars and (so called) health bars as I feel about protein- and slimming shakes - they are all 'dead' foods with hidden and hyped ingredients. 'Natural' colorings and flavorings are often questionable and so are the sweeteners. I would much rather eat an apple, orange, pear, peach or any other natural and satisfying snack. Fruit is also very cost effective!

HEALTHY BREAD AND CRACKERS

Most people are extremely misinformed when it comes to ‘healthy’ bread. The ingredients on bread labels should not be a lengthy list with unpronounceable words - they should be simple, for example, *"100% stoneground wholewheat flour, water, honey, salt, yeast"*. If the label states that it contains "sprouted wholewheat", then that would be a good choice as well.

Crackers are sadly misleading as well. The only store-bought crispbread or cracker I support is made with 100% rye. Homemade raw flax seed crackers made in a dehydrator is a good snack food.

Unhealthy bread and crackers that contain undesired ingredients, not only lead to weight gain, but painful joints as well, which in turn leads to the use of medications that have serious side effects.

THYROID DISORDERS

Medical practitioners are prescribing daily, to hundreds of people, mostly women, the ingestion of radioactive iodine (RAI). Patients are then prescribed synthetic or animal derived thyroid hormones, which needs to be taken orally on a daily basis to prevent death.

The thyroid gland is an endocrine gland and secretes hormones directly into the blood, which are essential to normal body growth in infancy and childhood. These hormones increase the rate of metabolism; affect body temperature; regulate protein, carbohydrate and fat catabolism in all cells; maintain growth hormone secretion; skeletal maturation; the cardiac rate, force and output; promote central nervous system development; stimulate the synthesis of many enzymes, and are necessary for muscle tone and vigor.

Disorders of the thyroid include Hyperthyroidism characterized by hyperactivity of the gland resulting in secreting larger than normal amounts of the thyroid hormones thyroxine and triiodothyronine accelerating the metabolic process of the body. Symptoms include nervousness, exophthalmos (protrusion of the eyeballs), tremor of the hands and tongue, ravenous appetite as a result of constant hunger accompanied by weight loss, fatigue, heat intolerance, palpitations and diarrhea. Untreated hyperthyroidism may lead to death due to cardiac failure.

Medically 3 different treatments are available:

1) **Thyroidectomy** - the complete or partial surgical removal (often 90 - 95%) of the thyroid gland. General anesthetic, hospitalization, stitches, sick leave and large medical bills result, and is therefore not the most popular treatment. In addition, the accidental removal of the parathyroid glands attached to the dorsal surfaces of the lateral lobes of the thyroid gland (behind the thyroid) may lead to tetany

(cramps, convulsions and twitching of muscles). The parathyroid glands secrete parathyroid hormone which assists in maintaining the level of blood calcium concentration and ensures normal neuromuscular irritability, blood clotting and cell membrane permeability.

2) **Anti-thyroid drugs** (propylthiouracil or methimazole) - Tablets may be prescribed according to the severity of the disorder. Side affects include rash, nausea, headaches and gastro-intestinal disturbances, agranulocytosis (reduction of granulocytes) resulting in bleeding ulcers of the rectum, mouth and vagina; alopecia (hair loss); thrombocytopenia (reduction or destruction of platelets resulting in bleeding disorders); aplastic anemia (a deficiency of all of the formed elements of the blood representing a failure of the cell-generating capacity of the bone marrow); hepatitis and psychotic reactions have been reported.

3) **Radioactive Iodine (RAI)** - the absorption and incorporation by the thyroid of RAI administered orally, rapidly absorbed by the stomach and concentrated in the thyroid. As iodine is absorbed by the thyroid gland, large doses permanently destroy the thyroid gland cells prohibiting the production and secretion of thyroid hormones thyroxine and triiodothyronine.

The treatment of RAI administered orally is most favored as it is rapid, effective and no recovery period is necessary. Any person receiving this treatment can immediately return to their daily activities.

With the treatment of RAI, most often all the thyroid gland cells are destroyed and if left untreated, will result in hypothyroidism - a condition characterized by decreased activity of the gland. Symptoms include weight gain, lowered heart rate and slowing down of the metabolic processes of the body, dry skin, alopecia (hair falling out), constipation, arthritis and cold intolerance.

Untreated hypothyroidism leads to myxedema (characterized by swelling of the hands, feet and face), coma and death.

Treatment for Hypothyroidism or the prevention thereof, is by administration of the deficient hormone. Pharmaceutical preparations of thyroid hormones are extracted from animal glands and the synthetic compounds levothyroxine sodium and liothyronine sodium are used as replacement therapy.

What patients who have medically had their thyroid destroyed and are on thyroid hormone replacement therapy do not realize, is that their lives depend on that one pill a day. Should they discontinue their life support tablet, they will slowly deteriorate into hypothyroidism, followed by myxoedema, coma and death within a few weeks. Are sufferers of hyperthyroidism informed of the drastic consequences attached to this treatment and that their life will, in future, depend on thyroid replacement hormones? Any person who has had their thyroid destroyed and is deprived of their medication (for whatever reason) will die. The majority of people are not aware of this very serious step when they ingest RAI. There are millions of people walking around without realizing that they are already on life support. Millions more will follow, totally ignorant of this knowledge. Are the effects of the treatment explained to patients? Are they warned that after the treatment they should stay 2-3 meters away from small children and infants for a period of at least 48 hours as they (the patient) are radioactive?

It is often claimed that the cause of hyper- and hypothyroidism is unknown but there is an enormous link between our food, metabolism and the thyroid. Incorrect nutrition is a major contributor, and a change in nutritional lifestyle can normalize the activity of the thyroid gland and avoid these drastic measures which threaten our life. Reverting to natural foods (fruit, salads, vegetables, grains, legumes) and eliminating the intake of refined and chemical foods (preservatives, additives, colorings and flavorings) could normalize homeostasis (natural balance or equilibrium) and return the body to optimal functioning.

CHAPTER 12
EATING DISORDERS

ANOREXIA NERVOSA

Anorexia is the loss of appetite, but anorexia nervosa is a symptom of anxiety neurosis, which is a serious disorder where food is rejected. Long term or permanent damage to the digestive and reproductive systems is common due to the lack of nutrients necessary for normal bodily functions. Amenorrhea, a common symptom in young women, can lead to infertility. Anorexia nervosa is damaging to the extreme and can sometimes be fatal.

Sufferers are obsessed with the idea that they are fat, and no amount of counseling will change their mental image. Often teasing from peers, pressure from parents or beautiful bodies projected by the media, triggered this.

Mental, physical and emotional healing is necessary for any person suffering from this disorder.

SYMPTOMS

- ❑ Finding reasons to be absent at mealtimes.
- ❑ Eating small portions.
- ❑ Playing with food.
- ❑ Looking 'busy' with food on the plate but not actually eating.
- ❑ Playing for time - taking a long time to eat a small bite.
- ❑ Denial of the situation or problem.
- ❑ Anger when questioned about (none) eating habits.
- ❑ Emotional and social withdrawals.
- ❑ Obsessive calorie counting.
- ❑ Fat obsessions - about being fat, and not eating fat.
- ❑ Laxative obsessions including diuretics, enemas, colonics.

MENTAL HEALING

Sufferers from Anorexia Nervosa must seek professional counseling from a qualified psychologist (or other professional) that will monitor them on an ongoing basis.

PHYSICAL HEALING

Nutrition is of the utmost importance as it provides the healing factor for the body, mind and spirit and is the only 'medicine' capable of repairing and restoring damaged bodily functions. Hippocrates (the father of medicine) said "therefore, let thy food be thy medicine".

It is recommended that nutritious foods and high quality 'live' supplements be introduced gradually under the guidance of a qualified and experienced naturopath and/or homeopath.

Protein is extremely valuable and necessary to assist the body in its healing and repair process. Animal protein is heavy and takes long to digest. Plant protein is lighter and digests quicker - not leaving the person with a full and heavy feeling. Hummus and bean dips with cucumber, squash and butternut slices (as chips) are nutritious, tasteful, digests rapidly, and are healthy proteins.

Fruit and vegetable drinks in the form of smoothies are nutritious, quickly digested, and are not weight-gain threats.

Frequent, natural food, snack meals are more recommended than 3 large meals per day, as the latter will leave a 'full' feeling and pose a weight-gain perception threat.

Lite natural food snack may consist of: fruit; natural organic yogurt and fresh fruit; salad; raw vegetable dips; smoothies; almond nuts and vegetable sticks.

Most definitely avoid man-made refined carbohydrates. These are real weight-gain threats that are addictive, and will do more harm than good for the sufferer.

High doses of zinc may assist in returning the sense of smell enabling them to smell and taste food. Zinc can be reduced and eventually discontinued when the appetite returns to normal.

EMOTIONAL HEALING

Self-healing is ultimately the key, but family and friends' love, understanding and patience, together with time, heal many unseen wounds.

BULIMIA NERVOSA

The same factors which prompt anorexics, prompt bulimics and range from lack of attention, poor self image, parental or spouse demands coupled with anxiety, stress and depression. Bulimics often binge, eating more than necessary because they are comfortable with the knowledge that they can rid their bodies of the food through purging or emetics (vomiting). Because of the fact that they eat well, they are socially camouflaged and their eating disorder remains unnoticed. Another reason why the disorder often remains undetected is the fact that many bulimics are older than and not as gaunt as the average anorexic, and often live alone or practice their bad habit in solitary conditions in the absence of their spouse or family.

SYMPTOMS

- ❏ Secret eating - hiding food or amounts being eaten.
- ❏ Eating large portions of food.
- ❏ Gulping food or eating rapidly.
- ❏ Guilt feelings about quantity eaten.
- ❏ Eating, even when not hungry.
- ❏ Lack of self-control with food.
- ❏ Expressing obsessive weight gaining fears.
- ❏ Laxative obsessions including diuretics, enemas, colonics.
- ❏ Discoloration of teeth caused by vomiting.
- ❏ Frequent bathroom visits.
- ❏ Disappearing after mealtimes.

Treatment rules remain the same for bulimics as for anorexics but fruit is the most bulimic friendly food as it is easily digested and nutrients rapidly absorbed into the blood stream before the sufferer has the opportunity to get rid of it through self-induced retching. A good source of natural 'live' multi-vitamins and minerals as well as high doses of zinc (as suggested for anorexics) is recommended for bulimics. Do not leave binge-eaters alone after a meal. Try to remain with them until the food has digested and absorbed by the body.

GUIDELINES FOR ANOREXIA AND BULIMIA

- ❑ Eat fruit - it is non-fattening and absorbed rapidly. It will not leave the person feeling full and bloated.
- ❑ Eat small meals fairly frequently (approximately three hourly). This too will prevent the person from feeling full and bloated. If desired, eat one food group at a time i.e. fruit; or a salad; or a small plate of vegetables.
- ❑ Avoid animal fat and protein. Eat plant protein often.
- ❑ Drink water as it is cleansing. Avoid diet drinks.
- ❑ Herbal tea is refreshing, non-fattening and alkaline forming.
- ❑ Liquidized fruit and vegetable juices are rich in valuable nutrients, and are rapidly absorbed by the circulatory system.
- ❑ Administer oral spray multi-vitamins and minerals. These are immediately absorbed into the blood stream and bypass the digestive system. Their organic nutrient content have the ability to normalize the digestive system.
- ❑ Ensure breakfast is a nourishing meal consisting of fruit, mixed nuts and unflavored yogurt with raw honey to sweeten if desired.
- ❑ Do not force the person to eat. Reasoning is better than force or threats.
- ❑ Food combining is important as it will prevent weight gain. (Refer to Food Combining charts at the end of Chapter 7)

CHAPTER 13
LIFESTYLE DIETS

VEGETARIAN

It is far healthier to concentrate on plant protein and avoid animal protein as much as possible, as the latter leads to heart and associated disorders. Animal protein is more compatible with our bodies in winter and cold weather and should only be eaten when there is nothing else to eat.

People choose to become vegetarians for many different reasons, which could include:

- ❏ Health hazards posed from excessive meat consumption.
- ❏ Health hazards posed from eating contaminated meat, such as mad cow's disease, salmonella and E. coli (Escherichia coli).
- ❏ Conditions under which animals are transported to slaughterhouses; and cruel treatments received there.
- ❏ Methods used to slaughter animals.
- ❏ In support of animal anti-cruelty movements.
- ❏ Inability to comply with the increased meat prices.
- ❏ Unacceptable feed given to animals and as a result, we become what **they** eat.

People are under the misconception that all vegetarians are healthy. Vegetarians are only as healthy as their diet. Many vegetarians are 'bread-tarians' with excessive intake of carbohydrate and dairy products, which result in obesity combined with digestive and skin disorders. A genuine vegetarian will not be obese, but follow a balanced diet high in vegetables, fruits, organic whole grains, pulses, nuts and seeds (all of these foods being excellent sources of protein) with limited amounts of organic cottage or feta cheese, unflavored yogurt, eggs and pure butter; and project health devoid of allergies, diabetes, coronary diseases, high blood pressure, digestive and rheumatic disorders.

There are different types of vegetarians. Some may consume cheese, milk, butter, eggs (dairy products), but refuse meat, poultry and fish. Others may follow the same diet but eat fish and refuse meat and poultry and occasionally eggs as well. It is a personal preference.

VEGAN

Vegans are people who will not eat animal meat or products including honey and yeast; wear animal leather or fur jackets, coats, belts, shoes, briefcase or suitcases or use animal byproducts such as feather dusters or 'shammy' (chamois leather) cloths.

It is stated that vegans lack vitamin B12, vitamin D and calcium in their diet. This can be especially detrimental to children following the vegan diet, as these are essential for the development of healthy bones and teeth. A deficiency will lead to stunted growth in children, osteoporosis, rickets and weak muscles with loss of control. Vitamin D is also required for calcium absorption. Vitamin B12 is necessary for red blood cell production, good digestion and a strong nervous system. Wakame (seaweed) is a good source of vitamin B12. The skin, in the presence of sunlight produces Vitamin D.

MACROBIOTIC

Macrobiotics is a new word to describe an ancient and traditional way of eating. In Greek *macros* means 'great' and *bios* means 'life'. Georges Ohsawa (Nyoiti Sakurazawa), a Japanese, was told as a teenager, by doctors of Western medicine, that he would not survive his condition of tuberculosis and gastric ulcers, and had only a few months to live. He would not accept their diagnosis and turned to Eastern medicine to seek healing by studying the concept of yin and yang (the unification of opposites). He developed a diet based on the theory that disease results when there is an imbalance in the diet of yin and yang foods. Following this principle, he cured himself, and nearly sixty years later, died in

1965 at the age of 74, after sharing his knowledge with people from all corners of the earth. The macrobiotic approach is based on a diet of mainly grains and vegetables, but specific foods may vary from country to country according to the food available. For instance, in Japan the diet could consist of rice, vegetables, miso (a fermented soy bean paste) and tamari (pure soy sauce), but in England it could be made up of wheat, oats, rice, vegetables with a little fish and fruit.

The food we eat is the single most powerful factor which will determine what we are and what we become, as we exist only from what we ingest and that is structured into our blood, flesh and bones. For this reason, the macrobiotic person adopts the macrobiotic diet as a lifestyle to achieve balance in life, enjoying health with happiness.

The following are a few characteristics of the macrobiotic diet:

- ❑ There are no large amounts of liquid consumed, as excess liquid leads to fatigue, placing strain on the kidneys, which in turn causes backache. Quality liquids are only consumed when thirsty.
- ❑ Foods eaten are those grown in the climate of that country and eaten in the season in which they grow. Salads in summer and vegetables in winter. Processed and canned foods containing chemicals are avoided. The digestive system is viewed as the only processing plant for the food.
- ❑ Coffee and spices are avoided.
- ❑ Animal meat and other animal products are generally avoided due to chemical and hormonal content, but left to the discretion of the individual. Fish, shellfish, fowl and natural cheeses are generally eaten by those who feel they have a need for animal foods.
- ❑ Potatoes, tomatoes, eggplants and peppers are classified as members of the nightshade family and are not eaten as they have been known to cause solanine poisoning. The Incas of Peru offered potatoes to the Spanish invaders

hoping to sabotage their conquest, but the latter took the produce back to Europe where they became popular and were cultivated in large quantities.

- ❑ Sugar is avoided whether brown, white or in the form of honey or molasses.
- ❑ Fruit is eaten occasionally.
- ❑ Unrefined sea salt is an important commodity and each individual is left to find their own balance. Emphasis is placed on unrefined sea salt as the manufactured varieties lack the natural trace elements and contain chemicals, which promote the free flow of salt.
- ❑ Tobacco and drugs or other stimulants are not used.

Grains are the basic food as they supply proteins, carbohydrates, vitamins and minerals and are comfortably digested. The eight main types of grains are: whole rice, whole wheat, buckwheat, rye, barley, corn (maize), oats and millet. Whole grains are preferred, as they require chewing, which is a very necessary action to maintain the strength and health of teeth. Refined grains are not only depleted in fiber and nutrients, but also deprive the digestive system (starting with the mouth) of this necessary action. Chewing and coating food well with saliva is very important in the first stages of digestion.

Dried beans and other legumes take a secondary role to grains and the most popular are: aduki beans (small red bean cultivated mainly in the east), blackeye beans, haricot beans, red wonder beans, mung beans, soy beans, blue imperial peas, marrow fat peas, chickpeas, green lentils.

Vegetables are organically grown and are used as an addition to meals based on grains. Methods of preparation include steaming, boiling, baking, sautéing, tempura (vegetables are covered in a flour and water batter and deep-fried), pickled or (occasionally) raw as a salad. Sesame seeds are used whole or in the form of salt (gomasio), or a spread (tahini), or as oil to sauté vegetables.

Sugar in all forms is discouraged, and honey or barley malt extract is recommended for those who seek more sweetness and are not satisfied with the natural sugars obtained from vegetables and occasional fruits. Because the earth, at one time, was all sea and is still mostly sea, and because the mineral constituents of our plasma closely correspond with the mineral constituents of the sea, seaweed forms part of the macrobiotic diet and should be eaten regularly. It is an excellent source of iodine and many other trace elements, and the following seaweeds form part of the diet: Agar-agar (Kanten), Bladderwrack (Kelp), Dule, Hiziki, Kombu, Laver (Noti) and Wakame.

Committed macrobiotic followers will have wild foods (vegetables or weeds), in their diet for various reasons. These may include: Thistle (cooked with mixed vegetables); Nettles (cooked as spinach or soup); Dandelion (in salads; or a coffee substitute); Fat Hen also know as Goosefoot and All Good (soups, sautéed, boiled with rice or dipped in batter and deep fried); Couch Grass (tea); Burdock (tempura; tea or coffee substitute).

Water is consumed only in response to thirst and avoided in the absence of thirst. Often 500ml of water per day is recommended. Certain foods such as curries, highly spiced or salty foods will create a thirst and should thus be controlled. Liquid is obtained from the foods eaten by chewing well, which in turn assists with digestion. An excessive fluid intake will not only cause the kidneys to work harder and contribute to fatigue and backache, but will also affect the natural water equilibrium within the body which is composed mostly of water. According to the yin and yang concept, yin is acid and yang is alkaline.

In summary, the macrobiotic diet consists mostly of whole grains, cooked vegetables, brown rice, miso, sea salt, and very little liquid, fruit, salad and animal protein. The diet is rich in vitamin B12 and enzymes but lacking in vitamin A and C, and is viewed by some as not ideal for children. I disagree with this opinion, as children's diet high in sugar and refined products is definitely not ideal, and the macrobiotic diet would be a vast improvement on the junk food eaten by most children.

CHAPTER 14

ALLERGIES
AND OTHER DIS-EASES RELATED TO A WEAKENED IMMUNE SYSTEM

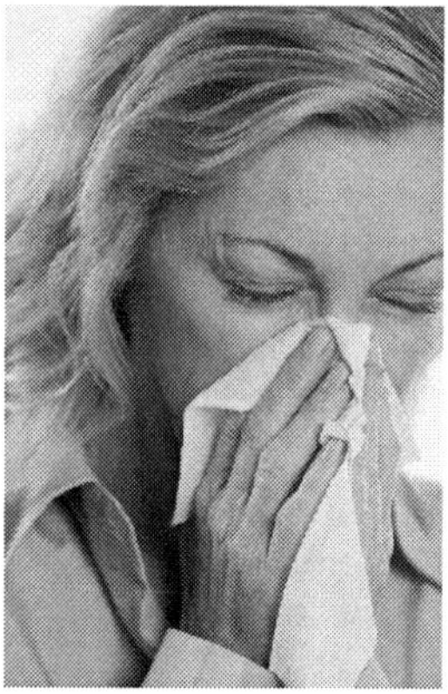

The body's defense mechanisms are collectively referred to as **immunity**. Derived from a Latin word, meaning 'safe', immunity is the ability to resist and overcome infection and disease.

Nonspecific defense mechanisms are adapted to prevent entrance of **pathogens** (disease-causing organisms), and destroy them quickly should they gain entry into the body. The skin is the body's first line of defense against pathogens and other harmful substances.

Specific immunity is needed when pathogens succeed in penetrating the body's barriers. Specific immunity depends upon the fact that each individual is biochemically unique. All human beings have some basic proteins, carbohydrates and nucleic acids, but just as no two individuals have identical fingerprints, so no two persons have identical macro-molecules.

During a lifetime people encounter different varieties of pathogens and build up specific immunity to them.

Although concentrating on allergy, and *Candida albicans,* **Diet # 6** given at the end of Chapter 15, is designed to **build up the immune system**. This is achieved by eliminating allergy causing foods (such as wheat, corn and soy) and food substances depleted in nutrients. The diet focuses on nature-made foods and will assist with the following complaints:

SYMPTOMS

- ❑ acidity
- ❑ arthritis
- ❑ asthma
- ❑ bloating
- ❑ bronchitis
- ❑ *Candida albicans*
- ❑ constipation
- ❑ diarrhea
- ❑ eczema
- ❑ fatigue
- ❑ flatulence
- ❑ hay fever
- ❑ headaches
- ❑ hives
- ❑ indigestion
- ❑ infections
- ❑ psoriasis
- ❑ sinus
- ❑ skin blemishes, rashes, itches and fungus
- ❑ urticaria
- ❑ warts and verrucae
- ❑ welts
- ❑ wheat or gluten intolerances

ALLERGIES AND THE IMMUNE SYSTEM

An **allergy** is an extremely sensitive reaction to harmless, mostly environmental, **allergens**.

Allergens are **substances** that are not normally harmful but cause a hypersensitive reaction in the body.

Substances are food, additives, pollen, grass, feces, dust mites, animal dander, animal hair, chemicals.

When babies are born, they live off the mother's immunities for the first six months. Their immune system is like a blank computer which needs to be programmed. The process starts when they make contact with foreign objects and place these in their mouths. They touch, feel, taste, and smell everything with which they come into contact. The brain appropriately registers the new data, and has the ability to call on this information at a later stage. As children grow, more information is programmed and the immune system is strengthened, or weakened accordingly if sufficient nutrients are not supplied.

The immune system is our defense system which fights infection and micro-organisms and aims to keep our bodies disease free. The immune system's function is to identify invaders and activate the body's white blood cells to act in response and phagocytose them (cell eating). The immune system does not have the ability to differentiate between a micro-organism and allergen substances as it merely acts on invasion. As a result, the immune system incorrectly identifies a non-toxic substance as an invader. Consequently, an alarm is raised and the body's white blood cells are activated to attack the 'foreign invaders'. This overreaction of the white blood cells causes more damage than the actual invader itself, which most often is a harmless substance. Consequently an allergy occurs when the body comes into contact, internally or externally, with a substance that is, under normal circumstances, not harmful but the immune system acts inappropriately in its response. The allergic response as a result becomes a disease in itself. These may manifest in the form of eczema, psoriasis, asthma, sinusitis, hay fever, urticaria and hives.

Any person, anywhere, can have an allergic reaction to substances. It very much depends on the country in which they live and substances common to that country. Wheat is one of the biggest culprits due to the overexposure to it in food sources. We consume wheat in the form of breakfast cereals and toast, sandwiches and rolls at lunch, pasta and pizza at dinner, cookies, crackers, pastries and cakes as snacks. Wheat is also used in processed foods as a filler. When the immune system is bombarded with a substance, because it cannot differentiate between friend or foe, it will react as though to invasion.

The first time a person comes into contact with a virus, such as chickenpox (measles, German measles.) the immune system is not certain whether it is friend or foe and whether it should allow it entry or attack it. By the time the immune system has realized it is foe, the virus has invaded the body. White blood cells will engulf the virus and phagacytose (eat) it. The characteristic blisters of chickenpox are confirmation that the immune system has won victory over the virus. Once the war has been fought and won, the white blood cells, which have acted in immune response, will guard the body against future invasions by calling on the now programmed memory cells. Before the virus will have the opportunity to invade the body again, memory cells will cause the defense to be called, and the virus will be destroyed before it can infect the body.

When T cells in the lymph nodes are sensitized and multiply, not all of them leave the lymph tissue and travel to the scene of the battle. Some remain behind as **memory cells**. Such cells apparently live on for many years and should the invading pathogen ever attack again, the memory cells initiate a far swifter reaction than occurred during the first invasion, destroying pathogens so rapidly that they usually do not have time to establish themselves, or to even cause symptoms of the disease. This explains why we usually do not become ill from the same type of infection more than once.

Exceptions are with conditions such as a cold or influenza as these are contracted more than once. The reason is that there are many varieties of these infections, each caused by a slightly different virus.

Furthermore, viruses frequently mutate, developing slightly different surface antigens in the process. Even a slight change can nonetheless prevent recognition by memory cells, requiring the body to treat each different antigen as a new immunological challenge.

The scenario is slightly different with food substances. Because the food source is consumed continually on a daily basis, the immune system (as it cannot differentiate between a food substance, fungi, bacteria or virus) will act as if it is being 'invaded' by the substance. As a result the white blood cells are continually active, unlike when the virus is annihilated and memory cells (T lymphocytes) protect against future invasions.

In these situations it is necessary to re-program the immune system. This is done by eliminating the problem-causing food (e.g. wheat or corn) from the diet for at least three months. Adhere to the Allergy Diet (# 6) as described in this book. It is imperative that there is no exposure to the 'causing factor' during this period of time, as it will allow the white blood cells to 'settle down' and give the immune system an opportunity to re-program itself. It is recommended that the allergy-causing substances are eliminated from the diet permanently but if, after three months, there is a need to return to these substances, they must be re-introduced into the diet slowly and in moderation as described in the diet.

FOODS LIKELY TO CAUSE ALLERGIC REACTIONS

These vary according to dietary habit. They are the foods most frequently consumed (in large quantities) and vary from country to country.

Most common: Wheat, soy, dairy, eggs.

Other common foods: Shellfish, nuts, peanuts, chocolate, citrus, tomatoes, berries, pork, beef, corn, peas, food dyes, colorings, additives, spices, e.g., cinnamon and nutmeg.

SYMPTOMS RELATED TO ALLERGIC IMBALANCES	
Chest:	Dry cough, breathing difficulties, wheezing, asthma, constant colds, nasal discharge.
Colon:	Irritable bowel syndrome, spastic colon, constipation, diarrhea, colic, flatulence.
Digestive tract:	Cramps, nausea, indigestion, bloating and 'movement' in the intestines, other gastro-intestinal problems.
Ears:	Partial deafness, fluid discharge, excessive wax secretions, ear infections, 'glue' ears.
Eyes:	Tears, itchiness, dryness, redness (both eyes), crusty lower rims or upper eye lids.
Nose:	Sneezing, itchy, stuffy or runny nose, post nasal drip.
Skeletal:	Joint pain in the ankles, knees, groin, wrists, elbows, shoulders, hips, jaw, arthritis and rheumatism.
Skin:	Rashes, itching, scaling, inflammation, blemishes, acne, pimples, blisters which 'pop' and peel, hives, eczema, psoriasis.
Throat:	Irritation, continual clearing of the throat, hay fever, sinusitis.
General conditions:	Headaches, food cravings, hunger, mood swings, emotional outbreaks, irritability, behavioral problems, hyperactivity and fatigue.

CHILDREN AND ALLERGIES

Children suffering from allergies are often pale, with runny or stuffy noses. They have dark circles under the eyes and their lids (especially lower) may be slightly swollen, and occasionally crusty. Often there are creases visible. Breathing is difficult due to stuffy noses, and consequently they breathe through their mouth. They are either hyperactive or hypoactive. Their coordination is often impaired and their concentration span is brief. Behavioral problems may fluctuate between mood swings, aggression and withdrawal. Headaches may be frequent, accompanied by slight vision imbalances. Often they will either not hear you speaking or not bother to listen or acknowledge they have heard you. Not all children are the same. Some may have only a few of these symptoms, while others may have many. Symptoms may appear immediately or days later.

DIAGNOSIS

Tests include the following:

Skin test - ingesting and inhalant allergens placed on skin may produce swelling.

Blood test sent to pathology laboratories.

Mucus - white blood cells may appear in the mucus of the nose, ears, chest, and stool.

Breathing and lung function.

CURE

Detoxification diet (# 4)

Eliminate allergy-causing foods from diet.

Maintain a healthy, nutrient rich, balanced diet. Follow Allergy Diet (# 6) for three months.

Build up the immune system. After the Allergy Diet, convert to the Acid/Alkaline Diet (# 3) for sustained health.

GENERAL ADVICE

When foods are eliminated from the diet, it is important to replace these with substitutes which will be equivalent and provide nutrients, e.g., replace wheat with other energy foods such as rye, barley, rice or potato flour. Brown rice, baked potatoes and maize meal (grits) are very good substitutes as well.

4-DAY ROTATION

Most important is a 4-day food rotation, especially with grains, legumes and nuts. When we study nature, food rotation in our seasons becomes obvious. Even within a season there are different food varieties - the list is endless but these are a few examples:

Apples - Galas, Fujis, Golden Delicious, Red Delicious, Granny Smith.

Avocados (almost 500 different varieties) - California Hass, Lamb Hass, Gwen, Reed, Bacon, Pinkerton, Fuerte, Zutano.

Potatoes - Russet, fingerlings, white, yellow, blue and red potatoes.

Onions - Vidalia, sweet, green, red, spring.

Nature in its wisdom knows that if we continually eat the same food, we will provoke our white blood cell activity, and provided us with seasons offering numerous varieties. Because of imports and refrigeration, seasons are no longer operative and the same foods are available throughout the year. It is now our responsibility, if we want to support a strong immune system, to eat varieties and prevent food sensitivities and allergies. For this reason a 4-day rotation is favorable where the same food type is not repeated within (at least) four days after consumption. This is especially important with grains to avoid **celiac disease**, which is an immune reaction to glutens.

Different grains such as amaranth, barley, buckwheat, corn, couscous, kamut, millet, oats, quinoa, rice and wheat are available with varieties within their species, e.g.: Rice: brown rice (long grain, short grain), black rice, basmati, wild rice - there are over 36000 varieties.

Wheat: Common (bread) wheat, hard and soft red wheat (winter or spring), hard and soft white wheat (winter or spring), durum, spelt.

If grain is required in the diet on a daily basis, then vary it: Eat oatmeal for breakfast; couscous at lunch and (herbal) wild rice at dinner. Do not repeat wheat at every meal – it is the quickest way to develop an allergy, or food sensitivity that will develop symptoms such as itchy skin, sinusitis or upper respiratory 'sniffles', headaches, fatigue, mood swings, red eyes, watering or flaking eyelids, painful joints (ankles, knees, hips, fingers, wrists, shoulders, jaw), irritable bowel syndrome, bloating, gas and mood swings. The old saying of "variety is the spice of life" is definitely applicable with our food consumption.

ALLERGY SUMMARY

- ❏ Build up a healthy immune system by eating fresh vegetables, salads and fruits. Vegetables are healing.
- ❏ Eliminate allergy causing factors, e.g. wheat, rice, corn, nuts, or other applicable factors such as chemicals, animal dander.
- ❏ Reprogram the immune system by abstaining from causing factors.
- ❏ Avoid eating the same foods repeatedly for lengthy periods.
- ❏ Adopt a 4-day rotation with food.
- ❏ Eat foods within their seasons.
- ❏ Remember: "Variety is the spice of life".

CHAPTER 15

CANDIDA ALBICANS

Candida albicans is a fungus or yeast organism, which is present along with many other micro-organisms in the gut of nearly all adults. Candida is an insidious yeast infection. It can strike anyone - even infants.

Most of the bacteria in our bowel are there for a purpose - to help digest food, to provide vitamins and to maintain the status quo inside our bowel. There are billions of healthy bacteria, which we are supposed to carry around with us such as:

- Lactobacillus acidophilus, Bifidobacterium bifidum
- Lactobacillus rhamnosus, Lactobacillus salivarius
- Lactobacillus plantarum, Bifidobacterium longum
- Lactobacillus casei, Lactococcus lactis,

The healthy population of lactobacilli in our bowel keeps the candida under control by competing with it for space. Antibiotics kill off dangerous germs as well as healthy lactobacilli.

Candida is an organism of low infectivity, but provided with the ideal environment, it will set up home in our bodies and cause many problems. As the candida multiplies we begin to suffer from the symptoms of yeast overload. Gradually our bodies accept the yeast as normal and give up fighting against it.

Candidiasis is the medical term used to describe the yeast fungus overgrowth. It is by no means a new medical problem; in fact, it has been around for centuries. Candidiasis has become a chronic modern medical dilemma that seems to be increasing rapidly. The reason for this is the declining vitality of many persons because of several generations of sub-optimal diets and the associated factors of drug and chemical exposure.

American doctor Orian Truss theorized *Candida* Hypersensitivity Syndrome in 1979. Controversy still surrounds the issue. His book *"The Missing Diagnosis"* was published in 1983.

FACTORS CONTRIBUTING TO CANDIDA

- ❑ Excessive use of antibiotics - especially of the tetracycline type. Candida 'eats' tetracycline antibiotic and thrives on it as a food source.

  If antibiotics are used, probiotics or any other form of acidophilus should be taken. Antifungal drugs should be used with tetracycline antibiotics.

  Consuming non-organic red meat leads to a further intake of antibiotics if hormones and drugs were administered to the beasts.

- ❑ Altered hormone levels: contraceptive pill, pregnancy and steroid drugs.
- ❑ History of taking cortisone (corticosteroids) - prescribed as an anti-inflammatory.
- ❑ Diet high in sugar - candy, cookies, cakes, breads, ice cream, sodas, commercial juices, pastries, pasta, pizza.
- ❑ Warmth; moisture - damp house or room.
- ❑ A weakened immune system.
- ❑ Hyperglycemia (a greater than normal amount of glucose in the blood) most frequently associated with diabetes mellitus.
- ❑ Chemotherapy, irradiation, prolonged illness, hyperalimentation (overfeeding, ingestion, administration of a greater than required amount of nutrients).
- ❑ Multiple food allergies and chemical sensitivities suggest that candidiasis may be active.

DIAGNOSIS

Although pus, stool, sputum, vaginal secretions can be smeared and stained on a glass slide and examined the same day for the presence or absence of fungal elements, there are no reliable tests, because if a swab was taken from inside anybody's bowel, Candida would be present.

Diagnosis is more usually based on symptoms, and often sugar cravings alone are a sure sign of yeast overgrowth. It is advised to follow the anti-candida diet, eating no carbohydrates for a period of two weeks up to three months, and closely monitor changes. Keep in mind this period could include withdrawal symptoms, which is an indication of being on the right track.

SYMPTOMS OF CANDIDA (not all are listed)

Candida symptoms manifests mentally as well as physically. Candia is a living organism, taking in nutrients and expelling waste the same as we and any other living organisms do. These toxins affect us in different organs and systems of the body. Severity of symptoms also varies from person to person.

MENTAL SYMPTOMS

anxiety	chronic fatigue	uncoordination
confusion	muddle-headedness	poor memory
irritability	mood swings	unexplained anger (emotion)
depression	lack of confidence	aggression (action)
self doubt	dislike of self and others	unexplained behavior

PHYSICAL SYMPTOMS

premenstrual bloating	nail fungal infections
cystitis	athlete's foot
acne	smelly feet
red, crusty eyelids	headaches
psoriasis and eczema	chemical sensitivities
urticaria	indigestion
skin rashes	heartburn
itchy skin	muscle & joint pain
skin 'blisters'	asthma
peeling, flaking skin	allergies
ringworm	insomnia
white (fungal) spots on arms and legs	lethargy
diarrhea	itching or burning in anus
constipation	low sperm count
spastic colon	prostatitis
irritable bowel syndrome	sexual difficulties
bad breath	infertility
frequent flatulence	vaginitis
foul smelling gas	vaginal or oral thrush

Other symptoms include:

- ❏ cravings: sugar, pickles, alcohol, sweet foods, bread
- ❏ Reaction to chemicals, fumes, perfumes, insecticides
- ❏ Water blisters on hands, fingers, underneath and sides of feet, which itch, pop and peel.

- ‘Movement’ in the intestines, especially for females. It gives the sensation of being pregnant, and often causes pain or discomfort and bloating.

Symptoms may worsen after eating bread, pasta, sweet foods, soy sauce, vinegar, or drinking alcohol. Symptoms are often worse in damp weather or a damp house.

In children the spectrum is different and the most common symptoms are behavioral: aggression, mood swings, tantrums, bed wetting and learning or concentration difficulties are sure signs of too much sugar, refined carbohydrates and chemical foods.

Often with babies, skin breakouts are mis-diagnosed as diaper rash. If the infant is breast fed, the mother needs to follow the anti-candida diet. For the infant, oral anti-fungal drops for internal use, and anti-fungal cream for external use, will relieve the 'diaper rash'. If the baby is old enough to eat solids, eliminate all forms of sugar and wheat from the diet and concentrate on fresh fruit and vegetables. (The same applies to the mother.) Do not give small children cookies, chips, cereals or other chemical foods to teethe on. Fruit or vegetables (such as cucumber sticks or thin apple wedges) are far more beneficial. Make certain they are not foods the child can choke on. Once children develop a 'sweet tooth', their immune system will suffer and other problems will set in. Refer to the Children's Diet (# 2) for further details.

Remember that children are building up their immunities, and refined, processed, chemical and 'dead' foods weaken their immune systems, which may result in allergies or food sensitivities, as well as behavioral problems.

Candida affects the gut and the rest of the body in two ways:

1) **The direct effect of the yeast:** Yeast fermenting in the gut causes bloating, gas and indigestion-type pains. Most often these conditions are diagnosed as irritable bowel syndrome, hiatus hernia or indigestion. They are mis-diagnosed, as the *Candida* is not recognized. Mis-diagnosis is also a direct cause of many unnecessary

surgeries that have been performed - yet original symptoms persist.

2) **Toxins and waste products produced by the yeast:** Candida produces toxic chemicals by its metabolism. All yeasts are designed to ferment sugars, and in so doing they produce alcohol and a number of other chemicals, such as acetaldehyde. This causes symptoms related to the brain and nervous system as well as the endocrine system.

WAYS OF FIGHTING *CANDIDA*

- ❑ Change your diet and starve the *Candida*.
- ❑ Repopulate the bowel with the normal bacteria or flora.
- ❑ Build up the immune system and restore it to its proper function.
- ❑ Minimize or eliminate immune-suppressive drugs and antibiotics - use only if absolutely necessary. These include cortisone (corticosteroids) and all forms of oral contraceptives. With the latter, affected women need to decide what is most suitable for them as it is a personal decision and unwanted pregnancies are not the aim nor solution. Following the Anti-*Candida* Diet would eliminate most problems experienced.

Besides dietary changes, there are other treatment methods dealing with candidiasis:

- ❑ Taking supplements to strengthen the body's immune system, and natural anti-fungal agents to kill the fungus.
- ❑ Taking anti-fungal drugs (most effective if done *with* change of diet).
- ❑ Colon cleansing.

NON-PERMITTED FOODS AND THE ANTI-CANDIDA DIET

A small percentage of **"no-no's"** or "not permitted" foods are allowed if it makes the difference between giving up and enduring.

I have studied and treated candidiasis for over 20 years and have found that if the diet is advised as strictly as stipulated in text books, people find it impossible to follow and consequently do not adhere to it, and then nothing is achieved. The first reaction from people is the comment "there is nothing left for me to eat". Most people who have been living on a diet high in refined foods and sugars have to be educated into the new way of eating. Agradual transition is often more effective and lasting than a drastic change, which in a short while, is going to be stopped anyway because people find it too difficult to follow. For that reason, I have allowed a few 'not permitted' foods in the diet for the sake of convenience and wider variety. Often these are the foods, which make the difference between people being able to continue, or not. It would be far more advantageous to those who are able to cope with their diet without these "no-no's". If not, these foods should be kept in MODERATION:

- ❑ ALCOHOL: This can be a problem for many people when mixing socially or entertaining. If an alcoholic drink *must* be consumed, have pure spirits (whiskey, vodka, gin or rum) with water in *moderation.* Avoid cola and other carbonated mixers or distilled water as well as wine and beer.

- ❑ ARTIFICIAL SWEETENERS: These are extremely harmful to the system and *should be avoided.* Those who are unable to go without sweeteners, rather use **raw brown sugar** (obtained from evaporated cane juice) in extreme moderation for a *limited period only*, to assist through the initial stages.

- ❑ CHEESE: Cottage, feta, goat's milk and small amounts of natural, unprocessed, uncolored cheeses. Occasionally a recipe may require a small amount of cheese. If kept in moderation, the system can tolerate it, if there are no allergies or lactose intolerance. Dairy products should be organic, hormone-free and used in moderation - especially while on the candida diet.

- ❑ FRUIT: The worst danger is getting hungry, as anything will then be eaten. If something quick, easy and simple to obtain (such as fruit) is not allowed, people opt for a cookie, chocolate or sandwich. I would rather people eat a fruit than a cookies, crackers or bread.

- ❑ 100% PURE FRUIT JUICES: for those who have a hard time giving up sodas. These beverages are depleted in nutritional value as they have been pasteurized and still have a high sugar content. They are also acid forming due to the process of boiling. For this reason, dilute with water and drink in moderation. Avoid grape juice for 4 - 6 weeks. The same applies to flavored mineral water. Although not perfectly healthy, I'd rather a person drink a small glass of diluted 100% pure fruit juice than a soda.

- ❑ GRAVIES: Use cornstarch (cornflour) as a thickener. Animal protein and gravy should be consumed in moderation.

- ❑ HERBAL COFFEE SUBSTITUTES as stocked by health food stores.

- ❑ HERBAL TEAS: Ideally, herbal tea should be fresh (from the garden) but if not available, use dried organic herb tea bags obtainable from stores.

- ❑ *RAW* HONEY OR *PURE* MAPLE SYRUP for those who *have* to sweeten. (Do not confuse pure maple syrup with ordinary syrup.) *Use sparingly.*

- ❑ CANNED FOOD: An occasional recipe may call for a canned ingredient. With candidiasis this is a 'no-no', but if 90% - 95% of the non-permitted foods have been eliminated, the canned ingredient (if not chemically laced) will be tolerated by the system. Again, these are small factors that could make a difference and encourage people to adhere to the diet thus obtaining the desired results, instead of discarding it because they find it too difficult to follow, and consequently experience no improvement.

I make allowance for the fact that we have been raised in, and live by, a 'convenience' lifestyle and that working mothers turn to convenience and fast foods. These foods are the culprits as there are not sufficient nutrients in packaged and processed foods - regardless of the fact that these foods have been 'enriched' with vitamins and minerals. Nonetheless, each individual has to take responsibility for their health and make a decision. If a person wants to improve their health and get well, **they need to make a concerted effort**. The immune system cannot be built up and health regained on processed, canned, frozen and packaged foods. Bear in mind that the recovery will only be as good as the effort made. If the diet is adhered to 60%, the recovery will only be 60%. If it is adhered to 100%, the recovery will be that much greater and the final rewards will be well worth it. My motto is, *"I never said it would be easy - only that it will be worth it!*

DIET TIME-PERIOD AND CANDIDA DIE-OFF

I suggest that the diet is followed for at least 3 months then SLOWLY introduce selected 'not permitted' foods back into the diet, but in moderation.

When commencing with the diet, '*Candida* die-off' (the fungus dying), may be experienced as well as withdrawal symptoms from certain foods. Headaches, fatigue, depression and a general feeling of ill health could result for 3 - 5 days and even up to 2 weeks. As described previously, I advise people to 'write off' the first 2 weeks and not expect major results. After that a reversed situation is experienced - feeling healthy, strong and energetic. Don't be misled into thinking that candidiasis has been mastered and discontinue the diet. The first symptoms to disappear are bloating, gas, 'movement' in the intestines, indigestion, heartburn, chest and abdominal pain as well as discomfort symptoms previously caused by 'spastic colon'. Next improvements with skin ailments, headaches, depression, anxiety, muddle-headedness and mood swings are experienced. After a month on the diet there will be definite and measurable improvement with many of the symptoms experienced previously.

If during the diet period there is a recurrence of candidiasis symptoms, or perhaps the desired results are not obtained, a re-evaluation of the diet is necessary to establish if any '*Candida* friendly' food is being consumed erroneously. Any “no-no's” should be eliminated and a more disciplined nutritional lifestyle adopted. It is important to realize that food tolerances and intolerances differ from person to person.

GUIDELINES FOR CHILDREN

(For a detailed list, refer to Diet # 2)

The same nutritional guidelines apply as for adults. Children are continually 'rewarded' or given 'special treats' such as candy, ice creams, cookies and other junk and chemical foods, causing them to developed a sweet tooth. Satisfy their sweet cravings with fruit - nutritionally that is the best food they can have.

It is virtually impossible to keep children completely away from candy, chocolates, desserts, ice cream, cake, pizzas, cereals and other junk food. For this reason, as previously explained, I have allowed a very small percentage of junk, convenience and other 'not permitted foods'. These include raw honey, raw brown sugar, unflavored chips, French fries, 100% pure fruit juices, organic wholegrain cold cereals, uncolored cheese, shelled nuts, raisins, 100% pure peanut butter, yeast spreads, and pure chocolates. Fortunately today, there are many foods previously labeled as junk that are now available in a much more healthy form i.e. organic ice-cream and organic pure chocolates. It is more acceptable to allow a child a small (more) healthy 'treat' than giving in to the normal junk food. From past experience, I have found that allowing a small amount of these foods, were the deciding factor with parents and children in adhering to, or discarding the diet. It is necessary to adopt a rule that when you have opted for convenience or junk food, giving the child a generous portion of fruit, salads or vegetables at another meal during the same day may make compensation. For example, if there are time constraints and your child has wholegrain cold cereal for breakfast, fruit should be eaten, preferably 20 minutes before the convenience food is consumed. Always avoid the exclusive consumption of 'dead' and nutrient depleted foods. It is difficult to expect a child to eat hot cereals (porridge) without sweetening it; thus the allowance of a little raw brown sugar is acceptable. The emphasis is on keeping it, and other 'not permitted' foods, to a minimum.

If all the 'not permitted' foods were eliminated from the diet, the situation would exist where mothers find it too difficult and restricting to cater for the children. Children feel too restricted as well. As a result, the diet will not be followed and both mother and child will achieve nothing. I do stress that chemical foods and beverages in any form must be kept out of the diet, as these weaken the immune system and allow Candida to flourish. Substitute *only* with organic, healthier similar types of foods such as commercial ice cream with organic types; commercial chocolates and candy with organic pure chocolates, commercial cookies and crackers with organic wholegrains.

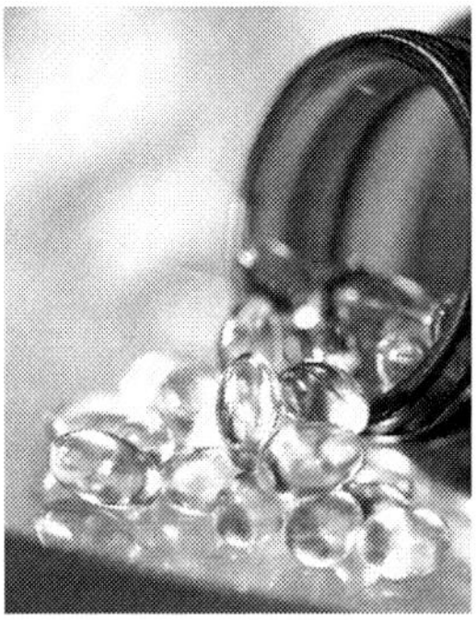

Optional: *'live'* multi-vitamin and mineral supplements (not synthetic vitamins), garlic and parsley capsules containing no colorings, flavorings or preservatives. Aloe vera juice and nutritious shakes, probiotics (acidophilus capsules or powder obtainable from health food stores). Although these are expensive and are optional, they may be beneficial in the initial stages.

ANTI-CANDIDA SUPPLEMENTS

Probiotics are 'good' bacteria that live in the gut and assist in fighting off hostile organisms. They are available in tablet or powder form. Acidophilus is a source of friendly intestinal bacteria and more effective than yogurt. Probiotics should be taken with oral antibiotics or after a bout of diarrhea. (Where possible, people suffering from candidiasis should not take antibiotics.) There are varied opinions as to when probiotics should be taken when antibiotics have been prescribed. My *personal* opinion is to take probiotics 2 weeks after the commencement of antibiotics and to continue until 2 weeks after completion of the antibiotic course.

Regular (not continuous) use of acidophilus culture keeps the intestines clean. It can eliminate bad breath caused by intestinal putrefaction, constipation, foul smelling flatulence, and aid in the treatment of acne and other skin problems.

Lactose, complex carbohydrates, pectin, vitamin C and roughage encourage additional growth of friendly intestinal flora. Friendly bacteria can die within five days unless they are continually supplied with some form of lactic acid or lactose, such as acidophilus. These supplements are expensive; eating organic live cultured yogurt often may help.

OTHER CANDIDA FIGHTERS:

- ❑ Garlic and clove - raw garlic or ground clove in food.
- ❑ Cold-pressed olive oil - contains oleic acid with antifungal properties.
- ❑ Aloe Vera (gel or juice) - have anti-fungal, anti-viral and anti-bacterial properties.
- ❑ Taheebo (also known as Pau d' Arco) herb tea - made from the inner bark of a Brazilian tree.

FURTHER YEAST OR CANDIDA FIGHTERS: coconut, nutmeg, cinnamon, linseed, sesame seeds, celery seeds, psyllium seeds, flaxseeds and liquid whey.

AROMATHERAPY OILS WITH ANTI-FUNGAL PROPERTIES:

Essential oils have similar properties but in varying degrees. Lavender, melissa, myrrh, patchouli tea-tree, sandalwood, cedarwood, cypress, lemon are a few oils with valuable antifungal properties.

Tea-tree is very effective, but do not use unless instructed by a professional, qualified in clinical or therapeutic aromatherapy. Health food stores, pharmacies and other store assistants are not always qualified aromatherapists and often their advice is inaccurate.

As a self-help for itchy, fungal or eczema skin, make the following blend:

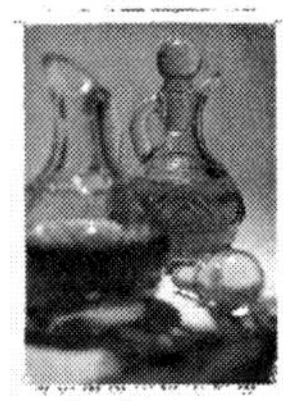

Lavender essential oil - 6 drops.

Tea tree (also called ti-tree) essential oil - 6 drops.

Lemon essential oil - 3 drops.

Olive oil (cold pressed, extra virgin) - 2 tablespoons.

Mix and store in a 1 ounce ultraviolet (UV) protected glass bottle (brown, blue, green, purple). Apply externally morning and evening (or as needed) to affected area.

NATURAL ANTIFUNGAL DRUGS (available from health food stores or homeopaths)

- ❑ Caprylate Plus - made from coconut milk.
- ❑ Paramicrocidin drops - made from grapefruit pips.
- ❑ Parquin capsules - in herbal form called Wormwood.
- ❑ Anti-Candida pilules – from qualified homeopaths.
- ❑ Caprilex tablets - contains caprylic acid which is a saturated fatty acid found naturally in coconuts.

(Not all homeopathic drugs are listed).

ANTI-CANDIDA DRUGS (Prescription only)

The purpose of anti-candida drugs is to kill the yeast. Most of these drugs are rather powerful and can kill the yeast very quickly. However, if a large volume of yeast exists, killing it off very quickly can cause extreme debility. It is recommended to diet for the first couple of weeks, avoiding refined carbohydrates, thus starving and destroying a large proportion of the candida before commencing with any of the drugs.

Many people experience symptoms of under-dosing, especially at the end of the first week. Symptoms include tiredness, headache, lethargy, depression and crying for no reason. The solution is to increase the dosage.

Overdosing is far less common but can occur. Symptoms vary, but include anxiety, jitteriness, feeling quite high, being unable to sleep and muscle twitching. Reduce your dosage.

Nystatin (Mycostatin): is an antifungal drug that causes the cell membrane of fungi to perforate, causing inner substance to leak out - thus killing the fungi. As with all drugs, side effects are listed with nystatin.

Nizoral is also an antifungal drug that works in a similar fashion to nystatin - it interferes with the development of the fungi membrane. When cell membranes are damaged, the cell dies as the function of the membrane is to keep desired substances within the cell and prevent undesired substances from entering. Unfortunately, amongst the many side affects of this drug, severe liver imbalances have been associated with Nizoral.

I foremost encourage candida sufferers to control their infection by following an improved lifestyle, which will starve the fungi and restore balance. Only in selected severe cases do I make a diagnostic referral for the treatment of extreme conditions.

Working closely with a medical doctor in South Africa who recognizes candidiasis, we found that the following prescription is more effective in the treatment of severe conditions:

- ❑ 1 Mycostatin tablet 3 times a day; 1 hour before a meal for the *1st and 2nd month.* This kills fungi inside the intestines.
- ❑ 1 probiotic capsule 3 times per day for the *2nd and 3rd month.* This replaces the friendly bacteria in the intestines and repopulates the bowel).
- ❑ Sporonox - although 1 tablet per month is normally prescribed, it is preferable if 1 tablet a day for *15 days* is prescribed in order to treat candida which has migrated outside the intestines into the tissue.

The reason we found this regime so effective was because Mycostatin destroyed fungi in the intestine while Sporonox destroyed fungi in the tissue. The probiotics, halfway through the treatment, started replacing good bacteria and repopulated the bowel.

In less severe cases a 1-month treatment is sufficient, but repeated if necessary for a second month. These treatments are expensive and must be done in combination with the diet. I recommend the treatment for a period of one month, and if symptoms persist, then continue for the second and perhaps third month. The above is merely one form of treatment - there are many, and individuals may wish to discuss them with their doctor, but the treatment described is definitely the most effective. Many doctors do not believe in candidiasis and will probably not agree.

Sufferers need **not** use the medication stipulated above as it has been given as a guideline only. A doctor may prefer Nizoral in place of Mycostatin, or Diflucan in place of Sporonox. I must emphasize that medications prescribed need to reach the **intestines** as well as the **tissue**, plus repopulate the **bowel** (as described above). Treatments will be ineffective if only one drug is prescribed to treat only one area, as in most conditions, candida infections are normally systemic (throughout the system).

There are many antifungal drugs available besides the ones discussed above. Individuals who desire to take this method of treatment are advised to discuss these with their healthcare professionalist (who recognize candidiasis outside the normal nail fungal and thrush conditions) and educate themselves with what is available (and most important) the expected side effects.

All drugs, natural or prescription, are expensive and if taken ***must be done in conjunction with the diet***. **Candidiasis can be controlled without the drugs by STRICTLY adhering to the diet,** as it has a two-fold purpose:

1) Destroy the fungus by means of starvation

2) Build up the immune system.

The fungus dies off relatively quickly but the purpose of following the diet for at least 3 months is to build up the immune system, thereby enabling it to recognize the fungus as foreign and suppress it.

For more information regarding *Candida albicans,* refer to books listed under Recommended Reading. Not all books are listed and further reading materials on this subject are available at bookstores.

KEEP *CANDIDA ALBICANS* UNDER CONTROL

Once the candidiasis is under control, care needs to be exercised with future nutrition and lifestyle. Concentrate on healthy food habits excluding, or keeping at a minimum, the factors that contribute to candidiasis over-growth. Maintain a strong immune system. After all, **you are what you eat.**

DIET # 6: ALLERGY, CANDIDA AND IMMUNE SYSTEM DIET

For people who suffer from headaches, fatigue, arthritis, wheat or gluten intolerance, candidiasis, gas, bloating, indigestion, constipation, diarrhea, skin rashes, infections, and allergies such as asthma, sinus, hay fever, bronchitis, eczema, psoriasis, urticaria, hives and welts - and for general good health to avoid disease forming conditions.

The following diet has been designed to detoxify the body, repopulate the bowel and build up the immune system. At first it may seem there is nothing to eat, but natural foods such as fruit, salads and vegetables are unlimited and may be eaten as much, and as often, as desired. It is advisable to eat small quality meals often rather than 3 large meals, as this will maintain correct blood sugar levels. Avoid getting hungry, as any food available will then be eaten.

This diet cuts out man-made foods and allows for nature-made foods. Man-made foods pollute our systems and are dead due to the chemicals used, the method of process, preservatives, the form of packaging and exposure to irradiation. These foods are produced, motivated by profit. Often, ingredients rendering the highest profit are used, and these are not necessarily the healthiest.

Nature-made foods are nutritionally balanced with vitamins, minerals, protein, carbohydrates, lecithin, fiber and liquids. These are for the benefit of the body to build up, energize, and revitalize the system, and keep it disease free and healthy. These foods detoxify instead of polluting the body. Compare eating a cookie with eating a carrot. A carrot provides fiber, vitamins, minerals, quality liquid, energy and works for the body. A cookie, apart from satisfying the taste buds, will do nothing except 'clog' and pollute body systems, and the body will have to use energy to eliminate it. Chemicals, additives, preservatives and flavorings used in these dead and processed foods will weaken the immune system and cause permanent damage over the years. *We literally eat ourselves to death on man-made foods.*

Due to its importance, I reiterate the following. The decision of whether or not to follow the recommended guidelines is personal. The desired results will only be achieved if the diet is adhered to. If the guidelines are followed 100%, the desired benefits will be achieved. If not, the benefits will equal the efforts made. In other words, if the diet is followed 50%, only half the benefits will be reaped. The choice is the individuals'.

Bear in mind that when the diet is implemented, the body begins a cleansing and detoxifying program. It is normal to feel considerably worse before there is improvement. Symptoms are tiredness, headaches, muscular and joint aches, stronger smelling and darker in color urine as well as bowel movements, emotional outbreaks and mood swings. This could last for 3-5 days or up to 2 weeks - improving daily. **Do not be deceived into believing that the diet is causing the illness.** It is in fact confirmation that it is working and detoxification has begun. The toxins being released are causing the debility.

I suggest the first 2 weeks are 'written off' and no vast changes are expected. Thereafter an improvement will be experienced which may include a feeling of well being, energy, clearness of mind, emotional stability and general revitalization. Each individual is different and reacts or responds accordingly. Monitor any progress made and see the changes. Take note of how the skin color improves as the body detoxifies - blemishes and other brown or white marks start to disappear. A weight loss will be experienced - first in pounds/kilograms then in inches/centimeters. Cellulite will diminish. Surely this is motivation enough!

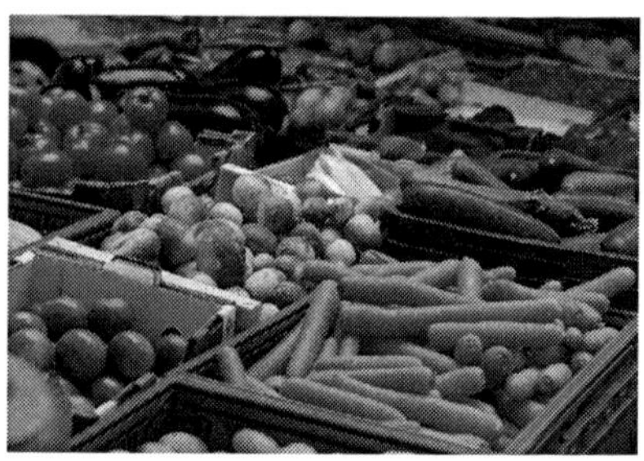

Should there be a recurrence of previous symptoms while on the diet, look at what has been eaten the last few hours or past two days. Certain 'not permitted' foods or liquids would have been consumed. Identify them and eliminate them from the diet to prevent future consumption. The first symptoms after consuming 'not permitted' foods will be bloating and flatulence - often foul smelling. Drink water often and eat juicy fruit to assist elimination. Prepare by reading through the diet, writing a shopping list, and then purchasing the items needed. Set a commencement date for as soon as possible, confirm self-determination to adhere to the diet in order to heal the body and improve health. Remember the diet is for *your* benefit and you are what you eat.

FOODS TO AVOID

SIMPLE CARBOHYDRATES/REFINED FOODS: white rice, pasta and all products made with flour and sugar - cookies, cakes, bread, bread rolls, pies, pizza, cereal bars. It is necessary to avoid all bread including whole wheat, rye bread and 'health' bread. Cereals, especially those containing sugar, bran and wheat.

ALCOHOL tinctures, cider, bitters, alcohol based medication ***(do not discontinue prescribed medications)*.**

PRESERVATIVES, COLORINGS, FLOVORINGS - All chemicals and ingredients that are unpronounceable.

SUGAR in all forms, and all foods containing sugar. Molasses, marmalade, jam, canned foods, cold cereals, canned or bottled drinks, candy, chocolates, cookies and cakes. Hidden sugar - read labels. Sugar may be listed as sucrose, fructose, lactose, glucose, maltose, dextrose and corn syrup.

YEAST, FERMENTED AND FUNGAL FOODS or drinks and mold foods include:

- ❑ Vinegar (cider, grape and malt vinegars).
- ❑ Soy products, soy sauce, tofu.
- ❑ Buttermilk, sour cream, cheese.

- ❏ Malted products (beverages, candy, dairy and cereal products which have been malted).
- ❏ Pistachio and other shelled nuts that are prone to mold. Natural oils in nuts go rancid when exposed to air.
- ❏ Dried fruit – prone to mold on the surface. Dried fruits are often coated with chemicals to make them shine.
- ❏ Mushrooms and truffles (a fleshy fungus).
- ❏ Canned or frozen citrus juices contain yeast. Freshly squeezed are yeast-free.
- ❏ Grapes have high sugar content and often have mold on the surface. Grapes may be introduced back into the diet after 4-6 weeks but wash thoroughly.
- ❏ Yeast is also in the form of bread, alcohol, pickles and mold (particularly moldy cheeses).
- ❏ Monosodium glutamate (MSG) is often yeast derivative.
- ❏ Artificial spices – contain too many chemicals.
- ❏ Left-over food and teas gather mold, especially black tea used for ice tea.
- ❏ Individual B-vitamins, B-complex vitamins, multi-vitamins, antibiotics and selenium are often yeast derivative or contain elements that are. In certain countries, unless stipulated on the label that they are yeast free, they normally contain yeast.

OTHER FOODS TO AVOID:

- ❏ Processed foods: hot dogs, hamburgers, sausages, lunch meats, corned beef, crumbed coated foods and fish sticks.
- ❏ Smoked meats and fish.
- ❏ Tomato products: tomato sauce, ketchup, barbecue sauces, basting sauces, salad dressings (use olive oil and lemon juice).

- ❑ Packet sauces or soups.
- ❑ Flavored and spiced fast foods.
- ❑ Horseradish, fish paste, chutney.
- ❑ Yeast based bread spreads, jams and marmalades.
- ❑ Muffins (including bran muffins).
- ❑ Ordinary tea and coffee, including decaffeinated coffee.

PERMITTED FOODS

COMPLEX CARBOHYDRATES: Whole grains, legumes, vegetables and fruit. Complex carbohydrate foods provide bulk in the diet, and will prevent drastic weight loss. Avoid hypoglycemia by eating complex carbohydrates (including fruits) upon rising and before going to bed (which should not be late!).

WHOLE GRAINS: Wild and brown rice, basmati rice, oats, barley, rye, quinoa, millet, maize and corn (popcorn). If gluten sensitive, avoid gluten-containing grains of which some are: wheat, rye, barley, kamut, spelt and oats (but oatbran and oatgerm are gluten free). Other gluten free foods are: Amaranth, arrowroot, beans, buckwheat, chickpea (garbanzo), corn, lentil, millet, nut flours, peas, pinto, potato, quinoa, rice, sorghum and sweet potato.

Keep gluten grains low, and use a varied mixture of other grains as mentioned above. Use chickpea flour, potato flour, sago flour, buckwheat (a cereal plant) and corn starch for gravies and baking.

LEGUMES/PULSES: Dried beans, peas, lentils, peanuts. Shelled nuts should be sold vacuum-packed.

FRESH VEGETABLES, SALADS, SPROUTS AND FRUITS: Eat as often as desired. The diet should consist of 70-80% of these foods, which are alkaline. At least 2 out of 3 meals per day should consist of this food group. Many books advise against fruit because of the high sugar content. Fruit is natural sugar, compatible with our body, and is the one food that is available almost anywhere that requires no preparation. It is quick and easy to obtain and it is better to eat a fruit when hungry (or thirsty) than eat or drink commercially prepared food. Fruit will only be a problem if eaten with simple carbohydrates, such as pasta or bread. This will cause a fermentation process in the gut. The fruit is not the problem - the pasta and breads are.

FATS: Cold-pressed organic oils - olive, sesame seed, avocado, wheatgerm and grapeseed. Organic butter *in moderation.*

DAIRY: Skimmed or low fat milk (if no dairy intolerance). Live cultured yogurt - contains lactobacillus similar to those necessary for repopulating the bowel.

Cheese in moderation - cottage, feta and goat's milk cheese. If no dairy allergies, uncolored cheese may be introduced after 4 - 6 weeks.

PROTEIN: Found in milk, yogurt, cheese, meat, poultry, eggs (cage-free), fish, nuts, seeds, pulses, whole grains, fruit and vegetables should all be organic. *Animal protein* should be eaten *in moderation* and *less in summer* than in winter or cold weather.

NUTS: Brazil, almond, hazel, pecan, cashew, macadamia. Nuts should be in season and preferably in their shells, otherwise there is a high risk of mold on the surface and rancidity of their natural oils.

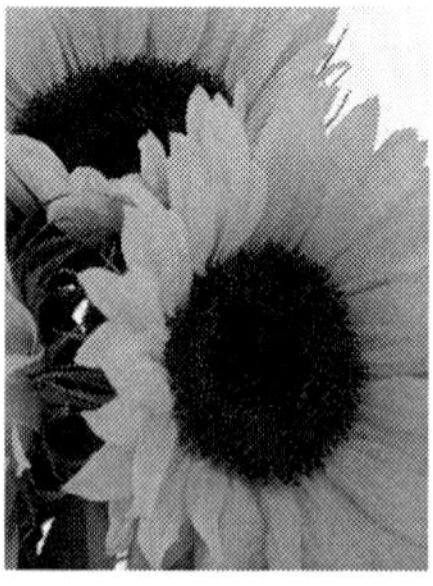

SEEDS: sunflower, sesame, pumpkin, linseed, chia.

TEA: Herbal (preferably fresh) otherwise organic dry herbs.

SUMMARY

PERMITTED

- ❑ Complex carbohydrates
- ❑ Whole grains
- ❑ Legumes/pulses
- ❑ Vegetables, salads, sprouts, fruit (in moderation)
- ❑ Natural fats
- ❑ Organic animal proteins and dairy in moderation
- ❑ Nuts
- ❑ Seeds
- ❑ Herbal teas

AVOID

- ❑ Simple carbohydrates/refined foods
- ❑ Alcohol, pickles, vinegars
- ❑ Preservatives, colorings, flavorings
- ❑ Sugar and sugar products
- ❑ Yeast, fermented and fungal foods
- ❑ Canned, frozen and partly prepared frozen foods.
- ❑ Processed, refined and smoked foods.
- ❑ Most 'man-made' foods.
- ❑ Concentrated frozen fruit juices
- ❑ Smoked meats and fish
- ❑ Commercial sauces and salad dressings

A more detailed guideline is supplied for those who require it:

NOT PERMITTED	**PERMITTED**
Dairy: Non-organic Margarine, butter spreads. Milk, flavored milk, buttermilk Yoghurt (flavored and colored). Sour cream Ice cream (commercial). Eggs in cartons Cheese (including moldy and processed).	Dairy: *Organic, hormone free - **in moderation** if no allergies or sensitivities*: Butter Milk (skimmed) Yoghurt (plain with live culture). Cream Ice cream (homemade - see recipe). Eggs - cage free Cheese: cottage, feta, goat, uncolored cheese.
Meat, poultry, pork, fish: Non-organic Sausages Processed (deli, sandwich) Canned Beef - corn fed and corn finished Chicken - caged Lamb that is not grass fed or grass finished Fish - farmed Pork - factory caged	Meat, poultry, pork, fish: *Organic, hormone free - **in moderation*** Venison and other wild game that are grass fed Canned (tuna, salmon, sardines) Beef - grass fed and grass finished Chicken - cage free Lamb - grass fed and grass finished Fish - wild or from deep ocean waters Pork - pasture raised
Grains: White rice, pasta, refined flour as well as refined products.	Grains: amaranth, barley, rice (brown and wild), couscous, flaxseed, millet, oats, quinoa, rye, spelt. (After 3 months organic wheat).

NOT PERMITTED	PERMITTED
Legumes: Soy and soy products. Sugar coated or flavored peanuts.	Legumes: dry beans, peas, lentils, raw peanuts.
Nuts: nuts with mold, sugar or too much salt	Nuts: almond hazel, pecan, Brazil, cashew, macadamia. Seeds: sunflower, sesame, pumpkin, chia.
Vegetables, salads, fruit and sprouts: Avoid canned or processed with added sugar. Do not heat or cook fruit Vegetable and fruit juices: Processed with added sugar and flavorings.	Vegetables, salads, fruit and sprouts: Eat any, all and often. ***Fresh*** before frozen, and frozen before canned. Vegetable and fruit juices: ***in moderation*** due to high sugar content. Freshly made, preferably with pulp.
Beverages: Fruit juices that are not 100%. Cordial concentrates. Frozen concentrates. Carbonated drinks. Tea and coffee Diet drinks. Milk based beverages (milk and orange juice, milkshakes, hot chocolate). Alcohol, tinctures, cider, bitters, alcohol based medication (do not discontinue medication prescribed by doctors).	Beverages: ***in moderation*** Avoid juices the first 4 - 6 weeks. Thereafter 100% pure fruit juices but dilute with filtered water to lower the fruit sugar content. If possible, try to avoid fruit juices completely. Herbal teas and herbal coffees Beverages: ***NOT in moderation*** Filtered water. Beverages: general Home-made almond milk - (see recipe)

NOT PERMITTED	PERMITTED
Cereals: Cold or hot cereals containing: Wheat, bran, sugar, colorings, flavorings, preservatives or other additives.	Cereals: Cold or hot cereals containing: Oat bran, oatmeal, maize meal (grits), sorghum porridge, granola/muesli.
Bread, crackers, cookies, pastries, cakes, pies: All wheat-based bread of any kind (read labels!). Bread rolls Pastries, pies and cakes Salty crackers. Cookies. Pizzas. Muffins	Bread, crackers, cookies, pastries, cakes, pies: Bread made from any flour that is **not wheat** and **does not contain wheat**. Cornbread. 100% Rye crackers. Rice cakes. Oatmeal-based pizza. Oatmeal cookie and oatmeal muffins.
Sugar: Avoid sugar in all its forms: Pure honey (heated and filtered). White or sticky brown sugar. Artificial maple syrup. SUGAR in all forms. Read labels for 'hidden' sugar, e.g., preservatives; flavorings in salad dressings, fish paste, chutney, sauces, jams, cakes, cookies, scones, bran muffins, candy, desserts, ice cream, chocolate, artificial sweeteners - the list is endless.	Sugar: ***in moderation***! Raw honey (unfiltered, unheated) Raw brown sugar 100% pure maple syrup

NOT PERMITTED	PERMITTED
Fermented food and drinks, yeast or mold foods: Grapes, pickles, soy sauce, mushrooms, vinegar.	Fresh lemon juice (in salad dressings in place of vinegar). After the system has detoxified apple cider vinegar or balsamic vinegar in moderation.
Commercial mayonnaise.	Home-made mayonnaise Store-bought grapeseed vegan-'naise'
Commercial salad dressings.	Home-made salad dressings (use olive oil, lemon juice and organic spices).
Instant packet soups.	Home-made soups.
Chemical seasonings.	Fresh or dried herbs and spices.
Candy, dried fruit containing preservatives and other chemicals which give them a gloss.	Fresh fruit, sun dried fruit and sultanas that contain no preservatives or any other chemicals.
Chips (all flavors) Popcorn (commercial and microwave) with butter, sugar or other artificial flavorings.	Chips (plain salted) very occasionally and in moderation Popcorn (home-made in dry popper). After popping, sprinkle with olive oil and herbal salt.

These are merely guidelines, as not all products can be listed. Fresh fruit, salad and vegetables are 'open' and may be consumed as much, and as often as desired. Avoid getting hungry, as anything will then be eaten. Snack on fruit or a baked potato, avocado, nuts, seeds. Refer to Acid/Alkaline Diet (# 3) snack list.

Optional: Multi-vitamin and mineral supplements (not synthetic vitamins) which are free of colorings, preservatives and yeast. Organic oral spray vitamins absorb directly into the bloodstream when sprayed into the buccal cavity, thus by-passing the digestive system.

SNACK MEALS: To maintain strength and avoid hypoglycemia, it is important to have 6-8 quality snack meals throughout the day in place of 3 normal meals per day. These snack meals should ideally consist of 'live' or 'wet' foods in the form of:

- ❑ Fruit, vegetables and salads eaten at approximately 2 hourly intervals.
- ❑ A baked or boiled potato is satisfying and may be used with various fillings.
- ❑ Celery, carrot or cucumber sticks with a cream cheese and yogurt dip.
- ❑ Tuna, chicken or egg salad.
- ❑ Brown rice salad consisting of brown rice with fresh diced vegetables such as cucumber, carrot, tomato, peas, celery with home-made mayonnaise or olive oil and lemon juice.
- ❑ Vegetable soup, stir-fries or casseroles are nourishing.
- ❑ Fruit, sunflower seeds or almonds are especially good when craving sweet things.
- ❑ Other quick snacks are rye crackers/snackbread or rice cakes with cream cheese and tomato, or a sliced boiled egg.

Followed this diet for at least 3 months. Preferably it should become a lifestyle, but any person who feels they cannot do without certain 'not permitted' foods, should slowly introduce these back into the diet, in moderation. These may include organic wholewheat and sprouted grain or seed bread (or any other 'health' bread), organic pasta and other organic whole grain products. Keep in mind that the more wheat products are avoided, the more beneficial it will be for our health.

The following counsel has been mentioned previously but I wish to reiterate my advice on wheat to those who feel it *has* to form part of their diet: when re-introducing wheat into the diet, do so gradually. Commence with once or twice a week only (e.g. Monday and Thursday), then three or four times a week (e.g.

Monday, Wednesday and Saturday). **Do not have wheat more than once a day.** For example: if toast or wheat cereal is eaten at breakfast, do not have sandwiches at lunch and pasta or pizza at dinner. If sandwiches or pizza is eaten at lunch, avoid further wheat products at breakfast or dinner, and should you know in advance pasta will be served for dinner, do not have wheat during the day. I STRESS THE IMPORTANCE OF LIMITING WHEAT INTAKE TO ONCE A DAY (OR LESS). The ideal situation is to eliminate wheat products entirely, but this is a personal decision. Alternatively, practice a 4-day grain rotation. Wheat today is not as wholesome as we believe it to be, and we would benefit more if we avoided it totally, or as much as possible. Remember: the whiter the bread - the sooner we're dead! This applies to *all* products made with refined flour, including whole wheat as it is actually refined. Attempt the diet for 3 months and it will prove accurate that wheat is a culprit contributing largely to many health imbalances.

If the diet has been followed successfully for 3 months and symptoms have cleared, and wheat products are re-introduced and symptoms manifest again, it is confirmation that gluten sensitivity exists. **If wheat or gluten sensitivity is experienced, then, unfortunately, there is no option but to eliminate it from the diet permanently.** As with Candida 'die-off', withdrawal symptoms from certain foods may be experienced when commencing the diet. Headaches, fatigue, depression and a general feeling of ill health could result for 3 - 5 days, and even up to 2 weeks. As advised previously, it is recommended to write off the first 2 weeks and not expect drastic changes. After that there should be considerable improvement with a reverse situation - feeling healthy, strong and energetic.

Alcohol is not a good idea at all but those who desire to drink should convert to pure spirits (vodka, gin, brandy and whisky) *in moderation.* Dilute these with water in place of sodas. Avoid wine and beer. For committed beer drinkers, German beer, or any other true brewed beer, is recommended, but must be consumed in moderation. Alcohol containing wheat should be avoided.

CHAPTER 16
GENETICALLY ENGINEERED (GE) FOODS

Genetically engineered (GE) and genetically modified organism (GMO) are words that have generated media interest. When we speak of GE substances, we refer to a process where genes are transplanted from one species to another, allowing cross-breeding which would never occur spontaneously in nature. Cross-pollination in nature has its limits, but GE allows modification across boundaries, which under normal circumstances, would never have occurred naturally. GE is dangerous, especially when animal genes are transplanted to vegetables and fruit. For example, genes from cold water arctic fish are transplanted into fruit and vegetables (strawberries and tomatoes) to prevent frost damage, and genes from insects are transferred to vegetables (potatoes) to protect against diseases. DNA injected is not limited to fish only - DNA of scorpion, spider, moth, mouse, chicken, virus, bacterium, animal and even human beings could also be used. Reasons given are that they:

- ❑ Increase resistance to disease: virus, moth, chicken DNA in potatoes and tomatoes.
- ❑ Increase resistance to insects: scorpion and virus DNA in cotton, tobacco, corn, rice and, tomatoes.
- ❑ Increase tolerance to herbicide: bacteria DNA in potatoes and corn.
- ❑ Increase tolerance to heavy metals: human DNA in potatoes and tomatoes.

This method of cross-breeding alters the characteristic and genetic structure of the new 'monster' food. The monster food does not have the ability to reproduce with seeds as nature intended, and basically 'self-destructs' at the end of a harvest, causing the farmers to purchase new seeds for each crop.

For years engineers have tried to justify the action of genetic engineering by claiming that this new method of producing substances will feed starving populations, limit disease (such as that caused by malaria mosquitoes), reduce the use of chemicals (pesticides), cause foods to last longer, taste better and crops to yield more.

GE foods are, unfortunately, not 100% compatible with our systems, as man is unable to reproduce what occurs spontaneously in nature. Furthermore, insufficient 'safety testing' has been performed, and sadly we have no proof of the long-term effects GE substances will have on our environment, or us. The environment is at risk as insect free cotton could have a devastating effect on our wildlife, as birds depend on insects as a vital food source. In addition, undesired cross-pollination may occur as wind, birds and insects carry GE seeds and pollen to organic fields, increasing the risk of these foods also becoming contaminated with GE genes. This could result in damage to our environment and ecosystem.

Many allergy-related conditions manifest when GE products are consumed, and clear up once these foods are removed from the diet. Insufficient time has been allowed to monitor and document imbalances caused by GE food. Allergies are not always linked to GE foods, but miraculously, these clear up once a wheat-free diet is adopted. In South Africa and USA, intolerance and allergy reactions are experienced with wheat, soy beans and corn. Unfortunately, many other countries are following suit with GE foods and these imbalances will spread. A large range of organic foods can still be found in Europe, as in 1991 Europe's organic farmers and processors decided that they would not allow genetically engineered materials in organic food production. For this reason, pasta and other wheat products imported from Europe are acceptable as they do not cause the characteristic symptoms of headache, post nasal drip, sinusitis, asthma, eczema, psoriasis, skin rashes and itches, mood swings or joint aches, which GE products may when ingested. In 1983 Europe's organic farmers also prohibited the feeding of meat to cows, thus preventing the effects of 'mad cow disease'. Japan use to ban GE foods. Unfortunately, many other developed countries, which previously did not support the concept of GE foods, are sadly, allowing genetic modification to take place. GE foods, without our knowledge, have very subtly crept into our diet (fresh and manufactured) and are continuing to increase on a daily basis. In South Africa, during the 1990's, it was estimated that 70% of products available on supermarket shelves contain GE ingredients. By now, that figure would have increased dramatically. GE products in South Africa can be found amongst fruits, vegetables (tomatoes, potatoes) and grains (maize, wheat and soy beans). Soy forms the basis of many processed meats, cereals, processed vegetarian foods, sauces, oils and infant formulas of which diaper rash is a direct result. South Africa imports large amounts of soy beans (also used as ingredients in bread, cereal and other products) from the United States, and more than 50% of that imported, is GE.

Edible vaccines, for humans and animals, which have been researched and developed for more than ten years, are a major concern as we are kept in the dark as to what is being fed to whom. Reported tests thus far are on mice, but where in the food chain do we fit? These edible vaccines are targeted for diabetes, hepatitis B, cholera, cancer, immune disorders and other human diseases. Bananas, tomatoes and potatoes are perfect foods for human edible vaccines. We are what we eat and we become what 'they' eat - so if corn, alfalfa and other plant foods become edible vaccine vessels for animals, by eating their flesh, we have yet another pathway to these vaccines. Hippocrates was centuries ahead of his time when he said *"Let thy food be thy medicine and thy medicine be thy food."* --Hippocrates (460-377 B.C.)

There is a vast amount of information available on this subject and many prominent media giants have written articles in an attempt to make us aware of the monster we are up against. We need to become pro-active and demand ingredients to be specified on labels. We further need to support stores that do not sell GE products, but offer organic products instead.

For further reading matter on the subject, refer to books listed under **Recommended Reading**.

CHAPTER 17
FOOD ADDITIVES

Introduction

What are additives? Additives usually have no nutritional value, and can be defined as a substance not normally consumed as a food by itself, or used as a typical ingredient in food. Additives, whether or not it has nutritional value, is intentionally added to (most often processed) food to enhance manufacturing processes, increasing preparation, packing, transporting and shelf-life expectancy of food.

There are more than five hundred additives that are commonly used in the commercial preparation of food. These can be divided into a number of groups as follows:

Colorings

Colorings primarily make food look more appealing, and thus more saleable. It is debatable whether they are necessary. Research has shown that bright and beautifully colored products attract consumers more readily than natural colors.

Many of the colors permitted are natural, such as chlorophyll, saffron, turmeric, sandalwood and paprika. This does not necessarily mean that they are problem-free. Most problems are experienced with azo and coal tar dyes which are black, brown, yellow, green and red colorants (everything except blue). These are potentially the most problematic.

The most notorious colorant is probably tartrazine. Much research has been done on tartrazine, proving both harmfulness and harmlessness. What seems to be most likely though is that nobody is allergic to tartrazine only. People with tartrazine allergies most often have an allergy to a foodstuff as well. Tartrazine also has a synergistic effect with the preservative sodium benzoate.

Preservatives

Arguably, preservatives could be beneficial, given the amount of food lost to spoilage, particularly in warm climates. However, there needs to be certainty that the benefits outweigh the risks. There are more than fifty preservatives, which are used in foodstuffs. Of these, eighteen are cited as causing problems. Whether the others are totally harmless is open to conjecture. However, it is questionable why the most dangerous preservatives are generally also the ones used most frequently.

Anti-oxidants

Anti-oxidants assist with the prevention of food spoilage, which occurs when in contact with oxygen. Foods which are particularly susceptible are oil- and fat-based foods. Some anti-oxidants are natural and benign, such as ascorbic acid or Vitamin C and Vitamin E, but others are seriously doubted with health questions attached, such as BHA and BHT.

Emulsifiers, stabilizers

Emulsifiers and stabilizers are used to stop ingredients from separating. Some, such as lecithin, are natural. Even this is not without its problems, as for cost reasons, lecithin is produced from soy beans, which could have consequences for people with soy bean allergies. Another reason for using these products is to get water to bind with processed meat, thus bulking the weight. Polyphosphates are usually used for this.

Sweeteners

Sugar, glucose and fructose are classified as foodstuffs; unfortunately, this category includes artificial sweeteners.

Solvents

These are used to extract or dissolve foods so they can be incorporated into products.

Anti-caking agents

These are added to powdered products, such as icing sugar and powdered milk to help them to flow freely and not stick together. Many of these products as relatively harmless as they are inert and not absorbed, but some of them could be problematic, such as talc.

Flavor enhancers

This includes some four thousand substances. The best known is monosodium glutamate (MSG). It is difficult to imagine any cogent argument for these additives, except for saleability of the inedible to the tastebud-challenged.

Mineral Hydrocarbons

These are used to prevent foods from drying out and as a polish to make foods shiny. They are used in dried fruit, candy, cheese rind and eggs.

Modified starches

These are bulking agents. Nothing much is known about their safety or lack thereof.

Miscellaneous

These are additives that nobody seems to know what to do with. Included here are propellants for food in aerosol tins, bulking and anti-foaming agents, acids, glazes and releasing agents.

There are also a number of ingredients that, although they cannot be classified as additives, are nevertheless secret ingredients in what we eat. These include fats and sugars.

Pesticides

Nowhere does a foodstuff have to show the amount of pesticide that it has absorbed on its way to the consumer's plate. Research report after research report shows pesticide to be carcinogenic. The most affected foods are wheat, potatoes, soy beans, beans, corn, tomatoes, lettuce, carrots, apples, peaches, oranges, grapes, beef, pork and chicken.

The law pertaining to chemicals

In European countries, 'E' numbers are a common sight on all packaging. An 'E' number is a list of additives that are supposedly regarded as being safe. They are placed on all foodstuffs that move in or around the EEC (European Economic Community) countries. Whether they are that safe, is a debatable point. Ingredients have to be listed in order of weight. This applies to South Africa as well.

Until a few years ago, 'E' numbers were never seen in countries like South Africa, except on imported foods however, with the devaluation of currency, more and more local firms are producing processed foods for the export market. In order to be able to enter the EEC, certain laws have to be complied with. This includes upgrading the amount of information given about ingredients using the 'E' numbers. EEC regulations are stricter than those in South Africa, therefore it is most revealing when reading the labels of foods intended for overseas markets.

Even in Europe there are still loopholes with declaring the contents of a foodstuff. Alcoholic drinks do not have to be labeled. Research has shown that by drinking two glasses of wine a day, one exceeds the acceptable safe limit of sulphur dioxide. Also, wine has to be clarified after fermentation. This can be done with many animal proteins such as gelatin, dried blood and milk proteins - a huge problem for vegetarians. Many beers not produced in Germany contain these and many more additives. Bread, confectionery and chocolate also fall through the loophole.

In assessing the safety (or 'unsafety') of additives, there are also a number of questions (besides the moral factors) surrounding animal testing. Accuracy is in question. For instance, tests on animal fed curcmin (an extract of turmeric) varied according to species. No adverse affects were seen in rats or mice, but the thyroid weight of pigs increased.

Food sold in South Africa needs no more than the vague term "flavor enhancer" or "emulsifier". Foods made under license to overseas multinational corporations are included. This makes it virtually impossible to find out exactly what ingredients are in a particular foodstuff.

The following present a sample of the amount of preservatives we eat on a daily basis in what many of us consider tobe a reasonably healthy diet. These are only the 57 additives that Hanssen considers being problematic and avoidable. The remaining five hundred-odd additives have not been included. It is necessary to note that possibly not all of the products contain all of the additives. However, some of them may contain additional additives not mentioned. Without proper labeling, it is impossible to ascertain.

Conclusion

There is a need for balance in this debate. It would be almost impossible to do away with additives completely, and possibly even unfair to poorer communities where refrigeration is a luxury. Thus there are compelling arguments for some. For instance, some preservatives are necessary to prevent illnesses such as botulism and salmonella, particularly for people who have no refrigeration. However, many of the processed foods that are preserved to death are in fact more expensive than their fresh counterparts.

Many additives do not appear to be damaging in the right quantities. Ideally, people should be re-educated into not believing that brighter food is better food. We can help ourselves by cutting down on processed food and avoiding the more unsafe additives. We can also empower ourselves by remembering that we control the purse strings and demand full and honest labeling. Labeling is of utmost importance for those who suffer with allergies, those who are looking for kosher, halal or vegetarian food, and simply those who want to eat as healthily as possible.

A day in the life of an average stomach

<u>BREAKFAST</u>

boxed cereal	*col* - calcium carbonate *anti-ox*- propyl gallate, BHT
yogurt	*col* - tartrazine, sunset yellow, carmoisine, *pres*- calcium sorbate, sorbic acid, potassium sorbate, benzoic acid, sodium propionate, sodium sulphite
orange juice	col- tartrazine, *pres*- sulphur dioxide, benzoic acid.
bacon	*pres*- sodium nitrite, potassium nitrite, sodium nitrate, potassium nitrate
eggs	*col*- xanthophyll *seal*- mineral hydrocarbons.
smoked kippers, haddock	
	col- tartrazine, quinoline yellow, kipper brown *flav*- liquid smoked flavor.
toast, bread, wheat products:	
	col- calcium carbonate, caramel *bleach*- chlorine, L-cysteine hydrochloride, potassium bromate, chlorine dioxide, azodicarbonamide. *emuls*- polyoxethylene stearate.
jam, marmalade	*col*- carbon black, sunset yellow, tartrazine, amaranth, carmoisine, red 2G *pres*- benzoic acid, sulphur dioxide, 4-hydroxybenzoates.
tea or coffee	*pres*- benzoic acid, 4-hydroxybenzoates.

cocoa	*col*- sunset yellow
	base- potassium hydroxide.
LUNCH	
packet soup	*col*- amaranth, ponceau, tartrazine, sunset yellow, carminic acid.
	pres- 4-hydroxybenzoates.
bread	see breakfast.
margarine	*pres*- potassium benzoate, benzoic acid, sodium benzoate
	anti-ox- propyl gallate, BHA
pickles	*col*- tartrazine, sunset yellow, caramel
	pres- benzoic acid, sodium benzoate
cottage cheese	*col*- titanium dioxide
cold meats, Vienna sausages	
	col- red 2g, erythrosine, ponceau, kipper brown
	pres- sodium nitrate, sodium nitrite, sulphur dioxide
mustard	*col*- tartrazine
DINNER	
meat, fish, sausage	*col*- red 2G
	pres- sodium nitrate, sodium nitrite, sulphur dioxide
	flav- MSG
stock, gravy powder	*anti-ox*- BHA, BHT
	col- carmoisine, amaranth, black PN, Green S
	flav- MSG
sauces	*col*- carmoisine, tartrazine, carminic acid, caramel, black PN

pres- sodium benzoate

flavored seasonings/salt

flav- MSG

salt substitute - potassium chloride

flav- monopotassium glutamate

herbs *pres-* sulphur dioxide

flav- MSG

stab- flour

vegetables - canned peas, beans

col- tartrazine, brilliant blue FCF, green S

flav- MSG

salad - tomatoes, carrots, lettuce

pesticides

olives *col-* erythrosine

pres- potassium benzoate, benzoic acid, sodium benzoate

mayonnaise, salad dressing

col- tartrazine, ponceau

pres- benzoic acid, sodium benzoate, 4-hydroxybenzoates

emuls- carageenan

chips *pres-* sodium hydrogen sulphite, sodium sulphite

bleach- potato white

ice cream, jelly, custard, packet desserts

col- carmoisine, amaranth, tartrazine, ponceau, black PN, erythrosine, green S, carbon black, caramel, carminic acid, quinoline yellow, sunset yellow

pres- sulphur dioxide, sodium benzoate,

benzoic acid, 4-hydroxybenzoates

flav-

emuls- carageenan

<u>SNACKS</u>

crackers *pres-* sodium propionate.

emuls- polyoxethylene stearate.

cheese *pres-* hexamine, sodium nitrate.

emuls- sodium lactate, carageenan, polyphosphates

candy *col-* carmoisine, tartrazine, sunset yellow, carminic acid, erythrosine, indigo carmine, caramel.

pres- sodium benzoate.

emuls- sodium lactate.

glazes- mineral hydrocarbons.

cookies, cakes, cake mixes, confectionary

col- erythrosine, indigo, carmine, caramel, tartrazine, carminic acid, amaranth, ponceau

pres- sodium propionate.

anti-ox- BHA

emuls- carageenan, polyoxethylene stearate

soft drinks *col-* tartrazine, caramel, red 2G, sunset yellow, carminic acid, caramel.

anti-ox- BHA.

pres- sodium benzoate, benzoic acid.

fruit *pres-* 2-hydroxybiphenyl, thiabendazole

sealant- mineral hydrocarbons

chips *col-* kipper brown.

anti-ox- propyl gallate.

	flav- monosodium glutamate (MSG).
raisins	anti-ox- BHA.
	sealant- mineral hydrocarbons.
chewing gum	*col*- tartrazine.
	flav-
	anti-cake- aluminum calcium silicate, talc.
	glaze- mineral hydrocarbons, refined micrcrystalline wax, dimethicone.

<u>DRINKS</u>

Tea, coffee	*pres*- benzoic acid, 4-hydroxybenzoates.
hot chocolate	*col*- sunset yellow
Wine	*col*- caramel
	pres- sulphur dioxide, sodium sulphite, CO^2, diammonium phosphate, ammonium sulphate, thiamine hydrochloride
	flav- diethylene glycol (antifreeze)
Beer	*col*- caramel
	pres- sodium sulphite, 4-hydroxybenzoates, benzoic acid, sulphur dioxide
	glazing- dimethicone
vitamins	*col*- amaranth
medicines	*col*- tartrazine
	glaze- refined microcrystalline wax
toothpaste	*col*- titanium dioxide

col-	**colorant**	***bleach-***	**bleaching agent**
anti-ox-	**anti-oxidant**	***emuls-***	**emulsifier**
pres-	**preservative**	***glaze-***	**glazes**
seal-	**sealant**	***stab-***	**stabilizer**
flav-	**flavorant**		

What is in the additive?

The following effects are the worst case scenarios. Not all of them happen to everybody. However, it is necessary to know what could happen.

Colorant	Effects
Aluminum (silver)	Has been linked to Alzheimer's. Used for dragées (cake decorations) only, so not likely to be eaten in large quantities.
Amaranth (red), Carmoisine (red), ponceau (red), quinoline (yellow), red 2G	Synthetic coal tar & azo dye. Adverse reactions in sensitive people and those with aspirin allergies or asthmatics.
Caramel (brown)	Can cause Vit. B6 deficiency
Carbon black (black)	Banned in USA, believed to be carcinogenic
Erythrosine (red)	As with amaranth. Also phototoxicity & can over stimulate thyroid production.
Indigo carmine (blue)	May cause nausea, vomiting, high BP, hypertension & allergic reactions.
Kipper brown (brown)	Two of the constituents cause genetic mutation.
Sunset yellow (yellow)	As with amaranth. Also gastric upset and urticaria.
Tartrazine (yellow)	As with amaranth. Also link with hyperactivity in children, particularly when combined with benzoic acid. Migraine, urticaria, rhinitis

Colorant continue	**Effects** continue
Carminic acid [cochineal] (red)	Linked with hyperactivity
Titanium dioxide (white)	Not harmful to the body, but mining is harmful to the environment
Patent blue V (blue)	Allergic reactions within minutes - urticaria, shock, breathing problems, nausea, low BP, hyperactivity
Brilliant blue FCF, Black PN	hyperactivity
Green S (acid brilliant green)	Slightly increased food intake, weight gain, anemia

Bleaching agents	**Effects**
Chlorine, Chlorine dioxide	Powerful irritant. Never shown to be safe. Destroys nutrients, esp. Vit E.
Potassium bromate	As with chlorine, including nausea, vomiting, gastric pain, diarrhea, convulsions.

Glazes	**Effects**
Mineral hydrocarbons	Chemically manufactured mineral derivatives for polishing, glazing, sealing. May result in anal seepage and irritation.
Refined Microcrystalline wax	Prepared from heavy fraction of petroleum. Carcinogenic.

Preservatives	Effects
Benzoic acid	Gastric irritation. Neurological disorders. Dangerous for asthmatics. Urticaria. Reacts with sodium bisulphite
Biphenyl	Produced by heating benzene. Nausea, vomiting, eye & nose irritation.
Calcium hydrogen sulphite, calcium sulphite, sodium sulphite	Gastric irritation. Thiamine destroyed. Dangerous to asthmatics.
4-hydroxybenzoates	Allergic reactions in asthmatics and urticaria sufferers. Skin sensitivity, numbing of the mouth.
Hexamine	Gastric, urinary tract irritation, skin rashes, gene mutation, carcinogenic.
Potassium nitrate	Gastroenteritis, vomiting, vertigo, muscle weakness, irregular pulse, can convert into nitrites
Potassium nitrite	Not for babies. Destroys red blood corpuscles. Causes asthma.
Potassium metabisulphite	Wheezing, cyanosis, faintness, unconsciousness in asthmatics.
Sodium benzoate, potassium benzoate, all sulphites	Allergic reactions in asthmatics and urticaria sufferers.
Sodium nitrate	Can convert into nitrites
Sodium nitrite	Nausea, vomiting, dizziness, blood deoxygenation, low blood pressure, circulatory system collapses, asthma.

Preservatives continue	**Effects** continue
Sodium propionate	Linked to certain migraine headaches.
Sulphur dioxide	Irritation of alimentary canal. Destroys Vit B. Dangerous to asthmatics
Sodium hydrogen bisulphite	Causes severe allergic reactions

Anti-oxidants	**Effects**
Butylated hydroxyanisole (BHA)	Raised lipid & cholesterol levels. Can break down important substances in body, e.g. Vit D. not for young children.
Butylated hydroxytoluene (BHT)	Rashes, increase in breakdown of important substances, reproductive failures, blood cell changes, behavioral effects, tumor formation. Not for young children.
Propyl gallate, octyl gallate, dodecyl gallate	Gastric irritation, reproductive failures, liver damage. Not for young children or asthmatics.
Calcium disodium EDTA	Used to bind with metal impurities in food. Too many could bind with body minerals.

Anti-caking agent	**Effects**
Aluminum sodium silicate, Aluminum calcium silicate	Aluminum has been shown to be neurotoxic, and has been linked with Alzheimer's, bone disease and kidney impairment.
Talc (French chalk)	Possibly linked with stomach cancer.

Emulsifiers, stabilizers	Effects
Sodium lactate	Could have a certain toxicity for young children.
Carrageenan	Ulcerative colitis. May be carcinogenic when degraded.
Polyoxethylene stearate	Some allergic skin reaction. May form kidney stones.
Polyphosphates	Could cause digestive disturbance by blocking some enzymes.
Potassium chloride	In large doses can cause intestinal ulceration. Sometimes nausea and vomiting.
Potassium hydroxide	Immediate burning pain in mouth, throat, stomach. Lining membranes swell & detach. Vomiting, pain & shock.

Flavor enhancers	Effects
Monosodium glutamate (MSG), L - glutamic acid	Heart palpitations, headaches, dizziness, muscle tightening, nausea, upper arm weakness, neck pains, migraine.
Monopotassium glutamate	Nausea, vomiting, diarrhea, abdominal cramps.
Calcium glutamate	Not for babies under 12 weeks
Disodium phosphate, Sodium 5' - ribonucleotide, Sodium guanylate	Avoid with gout

Bibliography

Hanssen, Maurice and Marsden, Jill comp. The new E for additives: The completely revised best-selling 'E' number guide. London, Thorsons, 1987. ISBN 0-7225-1150-7

CHAPTER 18
THE HISTORY OF CANNED FOOD

When reading about **Napoleon Bonaparte**, one would expect to learn about the history of a French artillery officer who rose to prominence and was appointed to command the French army in Italy, and not about the history of canned foods!

Napoleon devised a plan to conquer Egypt and India and break British imperial power. He successfully obtained the Directory's support.

Before he continued with his exploits abroad, Napoleon realized that by taking his soldiers on their campaign, they would need supplies which would consist of more that salted meat and fish. Like all sailors and soldiers, his army was affected by the lack of fresh fruit and vegetables, and suffered from related diseases such as scurvy.

He consulted with the Directory and requested quality field rations. The Directory realized the need and the enormous benefit of a solution, and consequently offered a reward of 12,000 francs to the person who could successfully invent a method to extend the lifespan of food by preserving it.

Lazzaro Spallanzani, born 1729, an Italian physiologist, was the first person to successfully perform artificial insemination. He did this by performing his experiment on a dog. He was also known for his studies of microscopic life and made it known to the world that the existence of spores in the air, and not the process of spontaneous generation, was responsible for micro-organisms.

Nicolas Appert, born 1750, was a French confectioner from Paris who became an inventor. He was familiar with the work of Spallanzani, and knew that in 1762 Spallanzani had found a way to prevent meat extracts from spoiling by heating them in a sealed flask. It took Appert fourteen years to perfect the art of preserving. He did this by filling glass jars with fruits, vegetables, meat, poultry, eggs, milk or cream. Leaving room for expansion caused by the heat, he sealed the jars with cork caps that were wired to prevent them from exploding off the jars.

In 1799 Napoleon returned to France and joined a conspiracy against the Directory. In 1804 he proclaimed himself emperor. Appert received his prize from Napoleon in January 1810, and in 1812 he opened the world's first commercial canning factory. Appert was described as the man who discovered the art of making the seasons stand still. Appert wrote a book giving an account on his work. "*The Book for All Households or The Art of Preserving Animal and Vegetable Substances for Many Years*" was published in 1810.

In 1810 further inventions were made to improve the process of preservation, and this time England's **Peter Durand** made a contribution by producing the first tin can. These tin cans were cut and soldered manually and the labor was time consuming. After food was inserted into the can through a small hole on the top of the can, the hole was sealed further by soldering a tin disc over it. Producing 50 cans per day, per worker, was considered very good and 60 cans per day was excellent production. People soon saw the value in this new method of storing and more and more canning factories opened. By 1840 these factories had spread internationally.

The next major contribution was made in 1860 by **Isaac Solomon**, a gentleman from Baltimore, the largest city in Maryland. Baltimore (with a population in excess of 786,755) is a major cultural and educational city and to this day boasts important industries such as steel, oil refining, sugar and food processing. Solomon discovered that by adding calcium chloride to the boiling water, the boiling point would rise from 212ºF to 240°F. This was a major breakthrough as it meant the processing time could be reduced to 45 minutes instead of the normal 6 hours. Production soared and factories producing 2,500 sealed cans per day could now increase their production to 20,000 per day. With this advancement followed other advancements. The can was redesigned to look similar to the cans available today. Larger lids allowed for larger sized foods to be canned.

During the 1820s canned foods in Europe spread countrywide, and by the 1840s it had reached the United States of America.

Not only did Napoleon have soldiers to contend with and solve a provision problem, but in America, they too were dealing with conflict. The Mexican war continued between 1846 - 1848. Five hundred men were called from a pioneer trail to form a battalion and go to Mexico to fight the Mexican War. So the invention in France, intended to nourish soldiers thousands of miles away from home, served the same purpose across the oceans for soldiers in other countries.

Canned foods were originally intended to save lives by supplying valuable nutrients when fresh food was not available. **We may benefit from this same principle if we eat canned food *only* when fresh food is not available.**

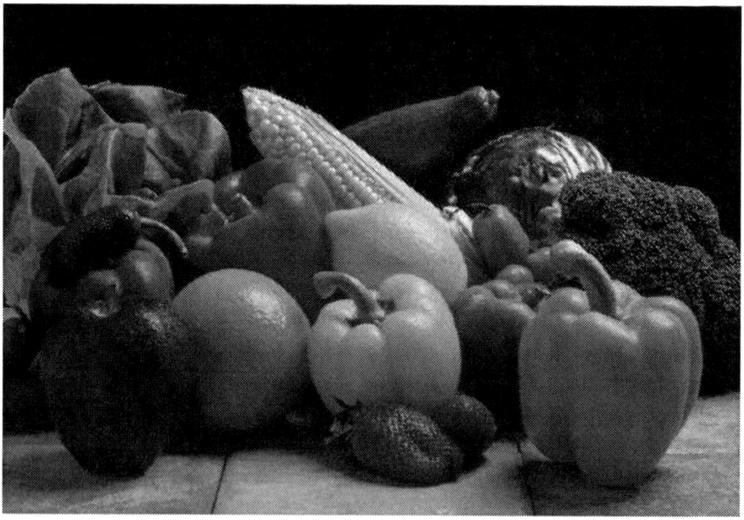

APPENDIX

RECIPES

The following recipes are mainly wheat-free, quick and easy, and the ingredients can literally be 'thrown' together. They are inclined to be dry, so increase milk quantities if necessary. Unfortunately, the baked items do not store long and dry out quickly. It is recommended to bake fresh often rather than store, but if baking in bulk, store excess in freezer. Gluten-free bread can be sliced and frozen, taken out when needed, defrosted, and either toasted or popped under the grill if soft and crumbly. Conventional recipes may be adapted to wheat-free ingredients by substituting wheat flour with oatmeal, corn flour, rice or potato flour. Refined white sugar can be replaced with raw honey or raw brown sugar. Animal ingredients (eggs, milk, cream butter, yoghurt, cheese) should be organic and hormone free.

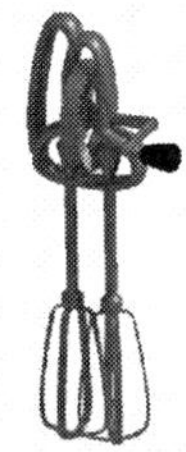

Abbreviation and Symbols		Pound - grams			Ounces - grams		
Kilogram	kg	2 lb	-	227g	¼oz	-	7g
gram	g	1 lb	-	45g	½oz	-	14g
milligram	mg	1.2 lb	-	700g	¾oz	-	21g
milliliter	ml	2 lb	-	907g	1oz	-	28g
pound	pd	3 lb	-	1360g	2oz	-	57g
once	oz	4 lb	-	1800g	3oz	-	85g
cup	c	5 lb	-	2250g	4oz	-	113g
Teaspoon	tsp				5oz	-	142g
tablespoon	Tbsp				6oz	-	170g
degrees Celsius	^{o}C				7oz	-	198g
degree Fahrenheit	^{o}F				8oz	-	227g
					9oz	-	255g
					10oz	-	284g
					11oz	-	312g
					12oz	-	340g

Cups - milliliters	**Spoon – milliliters**
⅛ cup - 30ml	¼ tsp (teaspoon) - 1ml
¼ cup - 60ml	½ tsp - 2.5ml
⅓ cup - 80ml	1 tsp - 5ml
½ cup - 125ml	2 tsp - 10ml
⅔ cup - 170ml	3 tsp - 15ml
¾ cup - 190ml	1 tsp (dessertspoon) - 10ml
1 cup - 250ml	1 Tbsp (tablespoon) - 12.5ml
2 cups - 500ml	
4 cups - 1 liter	

Oven Temperatures

Oven temp	(°F)	(°C)	Gas Stove
Very cool	200	100	1
Cool	250	120	2
Moderate	350	180	3
Moderate hot	375	190	4
Hot	425	220	6
Very hot	500	260	7- 8

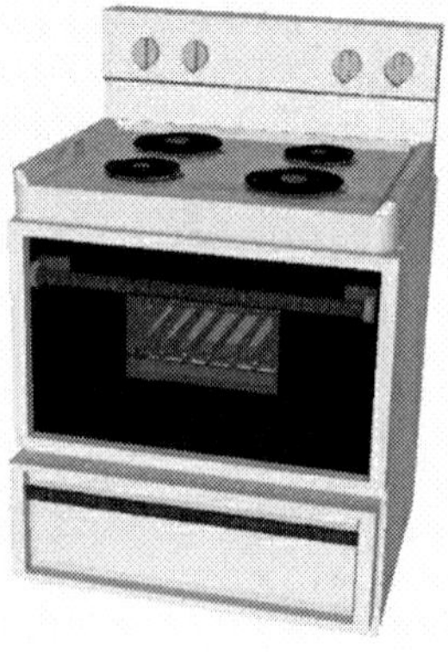

RECIPES INDEX

RAW FOOD RECIPES FOR BLENDER

(No cooking required)

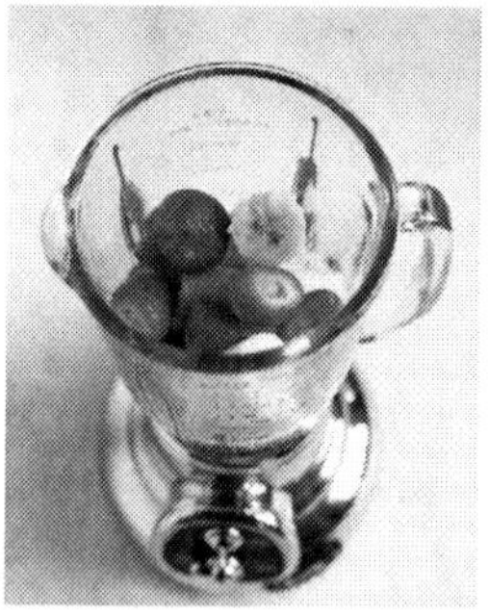

HEALTHY EATING - MADE EASY by Jessica Hart

RECIPES

ALMOND AND CASHEW SPREAD (in place of peanut butter)	
2 cup (raw) almonds	Salt to taste
2 cup cashew nuts	
1 Tbsp cold-pressed olive or any other cold pressed vegetable oil	
Combine nuts and grind until fine. Slowly add oil until paste is formed. Store in refrigerator.	

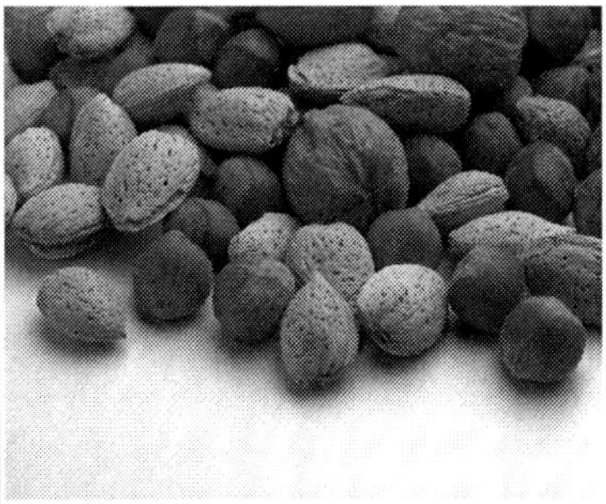

ALMOND MILK	
2 cups (raw) almonds	water for soaking
8 cups water	
2 Tablespoons raw honey (or sweetener of choice)	
1-2 teaspoons vanilla or coconut extract	

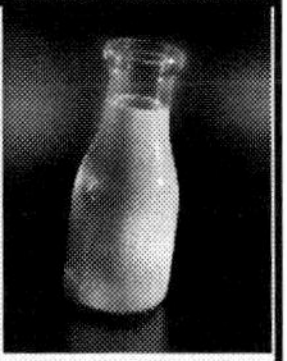

Cover almonds with sufficient water and soak for at least 4 hours. Discard water.
Place almonds in a blender with 4 cups of water and blend well.
Strain through a very fine strainer. Set almond milk aside.
Return almond pulp to the blender and blend again with the remaining 4 cups of water.
Strain and add almond milk to the milk set aside. Add 2 tablespoons honey or sweeten to taste with choice of sweetener.
Add *either* vanilla or coconut extract to taste (1-2 teaspoons).
Refrigerate almond milk in airtight container.
Pulp: use in smoothies or dehydrate (in dehydrator) for almond flour or discard.

BANANA FRITTERS	
1 cup potato flour	pinch of salt
3 mashed bananas	1 egg
1 cup corn flour	milk to mix
4 flat tsp baking powder	oil for frying
Sift dry ingredients together. Make hole in center, drop the egg in and stir to mix. Add bananas and mix well to a soft dropping consistency. Drop dessert spoonfuls of the mixture into hot oil. Fry until brown on both sides. Drain on absorbent paper.	

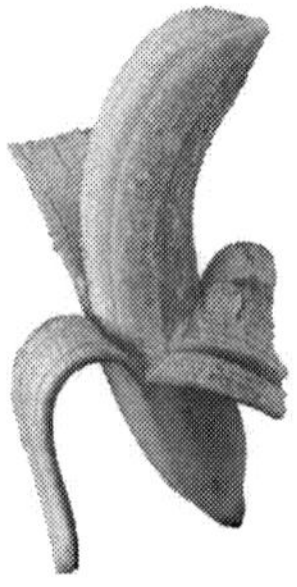

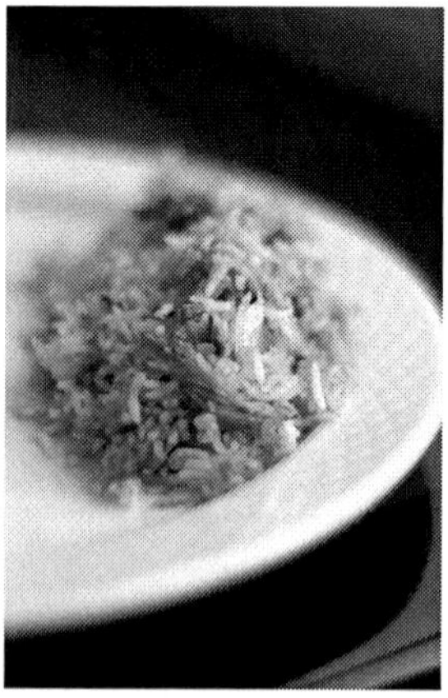

BROWN RICE SALAD
Boil 1 cup brown rice (or use left-over brown rice).
Mix in diced raw vegetables of your choice, e.g., carrots, cucumber, onion, celery, corn, peas, beans, cauliflower, broccoli, green/red pepper, etc.
Add 1 Tbsp cold-pressed olive oil, juice of ½ a lemon and herb seasoning.
Optional: crushed garlic or chili powder.
Serve warm or cold.

BROCCOLI BAKE (Serves 4-6)	
500g fresh (or frozen) broccoli, steamed chopped (optional)	30g (30ml) butter
250g rindless bacon	30g (or 1 Tbsp) corn flour / starch
2 fresh cloves of garlic, crushed	250ml cream
1 vegetable stock cube 100ml	250ml grated cheese
1-2 onions	3 large eggs, lightly beaten
250g mushrooms, chopped (optional)	
1 small green/red pepper, chopped (optional) boiling water	
Pre-heat oven to 140°C. Cook broccoli. Drain and arrange in an ovenproof dish. Fry onion, garlic, green/red pepper, mushrooms (and bacon) in sizzling butter until cooked. Sprinkle with corn flour. Stir in cream and stock cube dissolved in boiling water. Remove from heat and add the eggs and cheese. Pour sauce over the broccoli and bake for 45 minutes until bubbling and golden brown.	

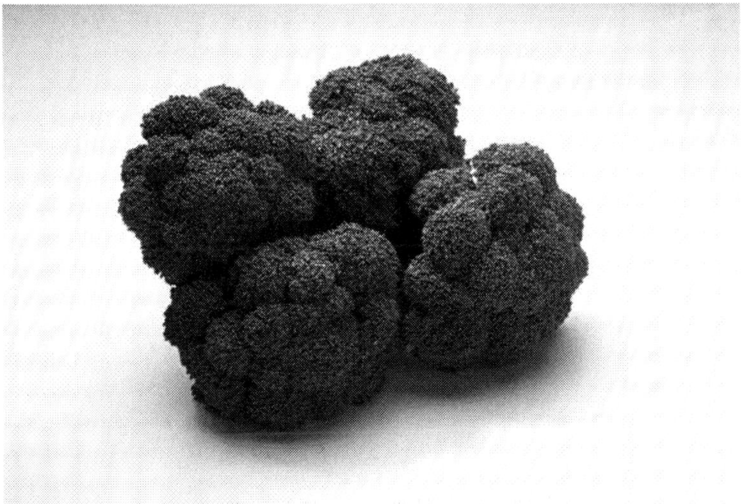

CAROB AND NUT / FRUIT / COCONUT CLUSTERS
Melt carob chunks (available from health food stores and looks like cooking chocolate) in double boiler. Add crushed nuts and / or sultanas (raisins) or coconut. Drop spoonfuls on grease-proof paper. Cool, and store in an airtight container.

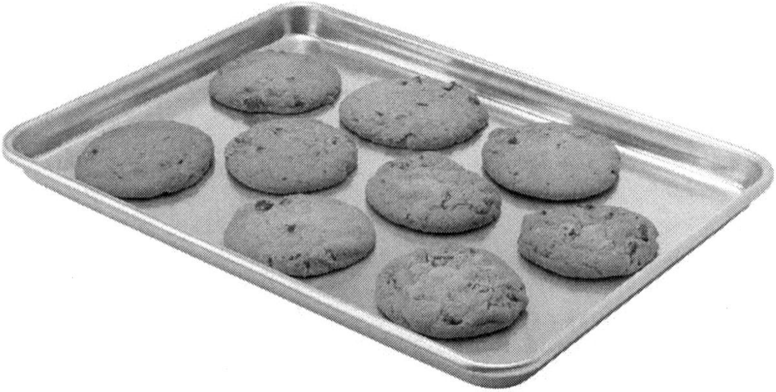

COOKIES (PLAIN)	
2 Tbsp butter	1 egg (beaten)
⅓ cup raw brown sugar	1 tsp baking powder
½ cup potato flour	a pinch of salt
½ cup corn flour / starch	¼ cup milk
Mix butter, sugar and egg. Add dry ingredients. Drop small spoonfuls onto a papered baking sheet. Bake at 190°C/375°F for 10 to 12 minutes.	

CORN BREAD (SAVOURY)	
1 cup corn flour	1 can creamed sweet corn
1 cup maize meal (grits)	2 eggs
1 tsp salt	¼ cup milk
2 tsp baking powder	
Grease container. Mix dry ingredients, add wet ingredients and stir with a spoon. Place in pan and bake in oven 180°C/350°F until light brown.	

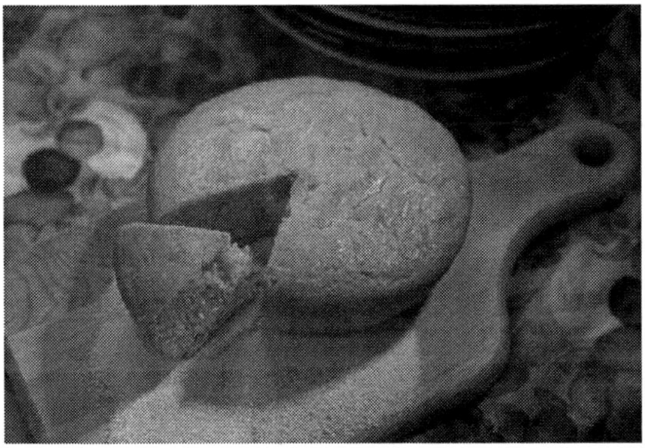

CORN BREAD (QUICK)	
1 cup maize meal (grits)	2 Tbsp butter
2 Tbsp raw brown sugar	125ml milk (half cup)
2 tsp baking powder	2 eggs
pinch of salt	
Melt butter, mix dry ingredients together; add melted butter, eggs and milk to dry ingredients. Mix well but do not over-beat. Pour into a lined loaf pan. Bake at 180°C/350°F for 40 minutes.	

COTTAGE CHEESE	
500ml buttermilk.	Tupperware Multi-serve
Line multi-serve strainer with cheesecloth. Pour half a cup boiling water in bottom section of multi-serve. Pour buttermilk into strainer section. Close lid and leave 8 hours or overnight. Separate cottage cheese from cloth and season to taste with herb or vegetable salt (optional).	

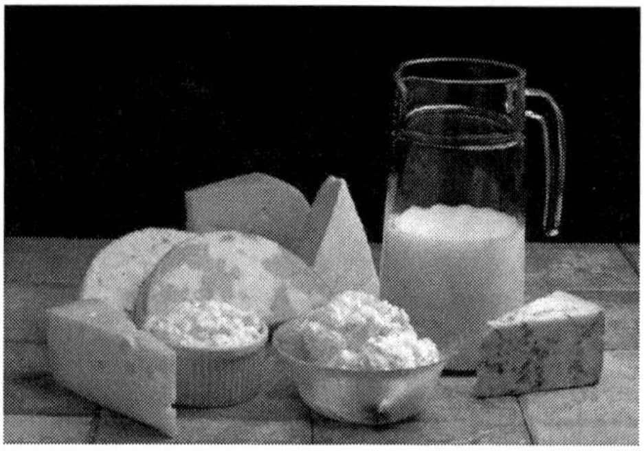

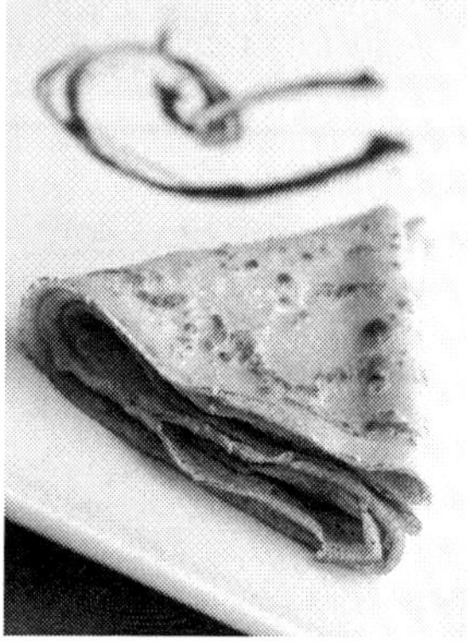

CREPES	
1 cup corn flour / starch	Cinnamon to taste
1 cup potato flour	2 eggs beaten
Water	¼ tsp salt
Make thin batter with flour, eggs and a little water. Add seasoning. Grease and heat a small frying pan. Put in sufficient batter (1 ladle) to cover the bottom of the pan. Cook until done on underside. Turn over and cook for approximately another minute (or until light brown)	

CRUNCHIES (a South African cereal cookie)	
500 ml oatmeal (not instant)	250 g organic butter
250 ml shredded coconut	15 ml raw honey
200 ml raw brown sugar	5 ml baking powder
250 ml flour	5 ml baking soda
Melt butter and honey in a pot on a low heat. Add baking soda and stir. Add remaining ingredients and mix well. Press into a greased baking sheet. Bake at 180°C /350°F for 25 minutes. Cut into squares while hot.	

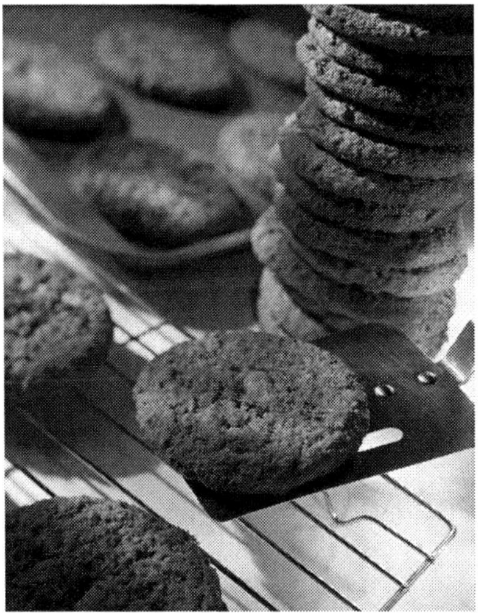

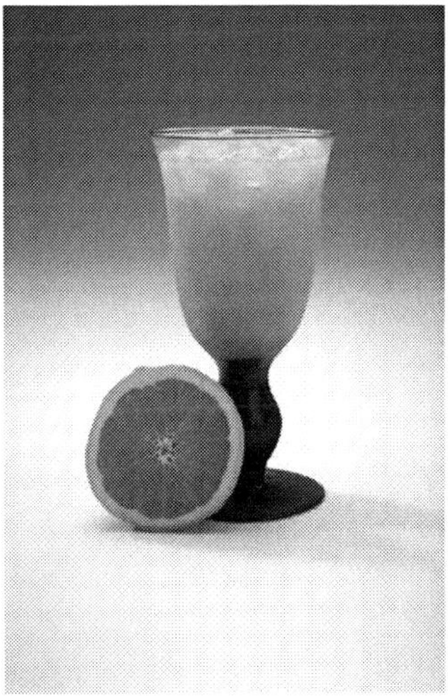

FLAVORED ORANGE WATER (makes 2 glasses)	
1 Orange	1 Tablespoon raw honey
1-2 slices of fresh ginger root (flavor to desired taste)	
1 glass water	Pinch of mixed spice (to taste)
Combine all ingredients in a blender and blend till smooth. Pour and add ice if desired.	

HERBAL TEAS (FRESH)
(all teas should steep for 5-10 minutes; strain and drink)
Ginger tea (aids digestion): Add 6-8 slices of fresh ginger to 1 cup hot water. Optional: Sweeten with raw honey to taste.
Lemongrass tea (skin tonic, headaches): Fold and snip one fresh leaf into pot, add boiling water. Optional: Sweeten with raw honey to taste.
Fennel tea (suppresses appetite, aids hormonal imbalances): Place 1-2 sprigs in 1 cup boiling water.
Parsley tea (detoxifies): Place 2 sprigs in 1 cup boiling water.
Mint tea (aids digestion): Place 2 leaves in 1 cup boiling water.

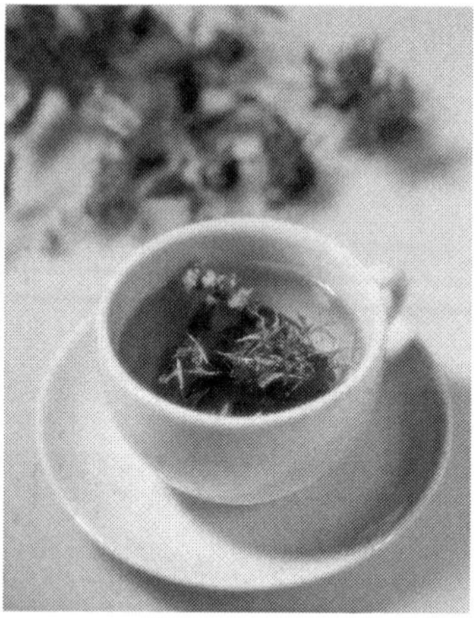

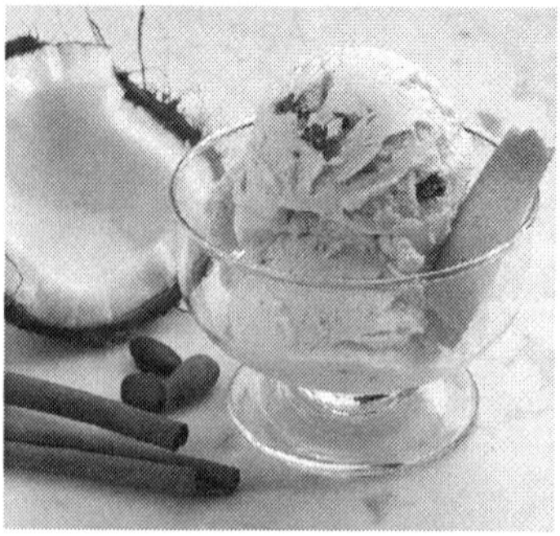

ICE CREAM	
2 bananas	2 Tbsp raw honey (or to taste)
*Frozen strawberries (be generous)	
Combine all ingredients in a blender and blend. *If fresh strawberries are used, add ice as well. *Frozen berries may also be used as an alternative Optional: Add nuts or coconut as a variation.	

GRANOLA / MUESLI BARS	
1 cup desiccated coconut	1 cup unsalted peanuts
1 cup sesame seeds	1 cup raw oatmeal
1½ cup sunflower seeds	
Mix the above dry ingredients together and place aside.	
Melt the following in saucepan on the stovetop stirring well.	
125g butter	¼ cup honey
½ cup brown sugar	
Add melted ingredients to the dry ingredients. Stir well. Spread evenly in a 20cm x 30cm pan, press down firmly with a cup. Bake in 350˚F/180˚C until golden brown. Slice into bars while warm. Leave to cool.	

GRANOLA / MUESLI	
500g rolled oats	1 cup sunflower seeds
1 cup light or dark sultanas (raisins)	1 cup sesame seeds
1 cup crushed nuts (Brazil, almonds, pecan, cashew - your preference).	
1 cup sun dried fruit (sliced or cut with scissors)	
Mix together. Prior to serving add sliced fresh fruit, milk or live cultured yogurt and honey to sweeten (optional).	

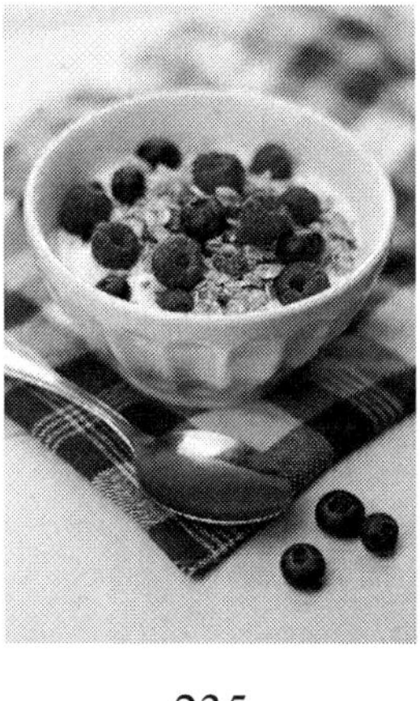

OATMEAL BANANA BREAD	
Dry ingredients:	**Wet ingredients:**
½ cup corn flour	2 eggs
2 cups oatmeal	1 cup milk
2 tsp baking powder	4 bananas
1 tsp salt	
sunflower seeds (optional)	
Mix dry ingredients together. Liquidize wet ingredients and add to dry ingredients. Grease container, pour mixture in and bake in oven 180°C/350°F until light brown. If the bread is dry, increase the milk or adjust recipe accordingly.	

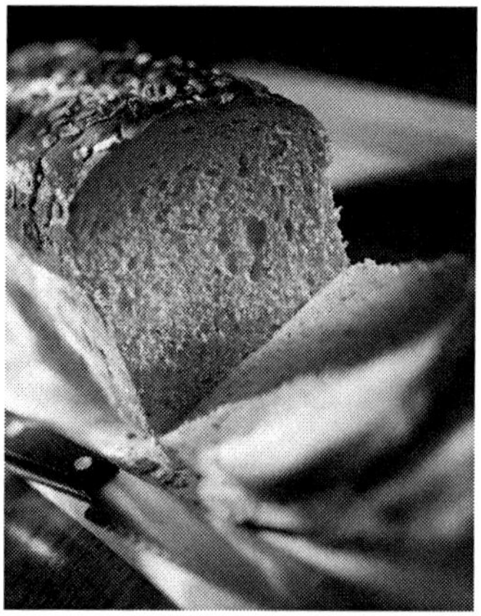

OAT BRAN SCONES	
1 cups oatmeal	1 tsp cinnamon
1 tsp salt	2 tsp baking powder
1 cup milk	2 eggs
1 cup oat bran (or grind oatmeal to flour consistency)	
1 cup mixed fruit: dates, nuts, apples, etc.	
Combine all ingredients with a spoon. Grease muffin tin. Spoon in and bake for 15 minutes or until baked at 180°C/350°F.	

OAT AND CHEESE SCONES (Makes 24 scones)	
2 cups oatmeal	½ cup corn flour / corn starch
1 tsp salt	2 tsp baking powder
2 eggs	½ cup milk
1 cup grated uncolored cheese	
Combine all ingredients and mix with a spoon. Grease muffin tin, spoon in and bake for 15 minutes or until golden brown at 180°C/350°F.	

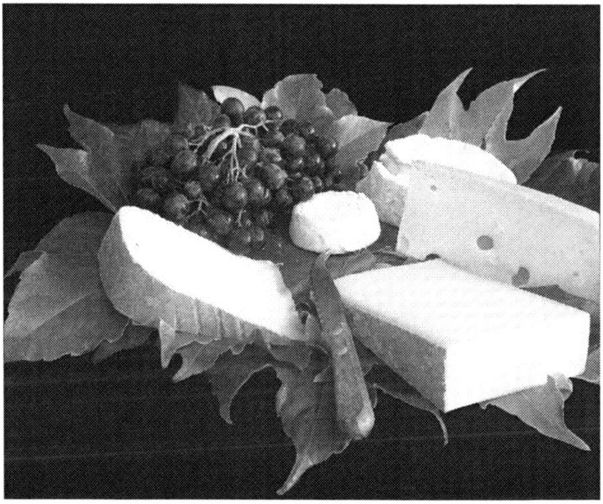

OATMEAL COOKIES (Makes 24 cookies)	
2 cups oatmeal	½ cup corn flour / starch
1 tsp salt	2 tsp baking powder
2 eggs	½ cup milk
½ cup raw brown sugar	
Optional: add sesame and sunflower seeds or desiccated coconut.	
Combine all ingredients and mix together with a spoon. Grease muffin tin. Spoon in mixture and bake for 15 minutes or until baked at 180°C/350°F. Spread onto a baking tray; cut with a knife when baked.	

PIZZA
Use the oat and cheese scone recipe above. Spread onto flat baking tray (spread with a tablespoon - dipping the spoon into a little milk **or** water periodically will make the spreading easier). Spread tomato paste on top of the base. Sprinkle with filling of your choice and grated uncolored cheese. Bake 180°C/350°F for 10-15 minutes.

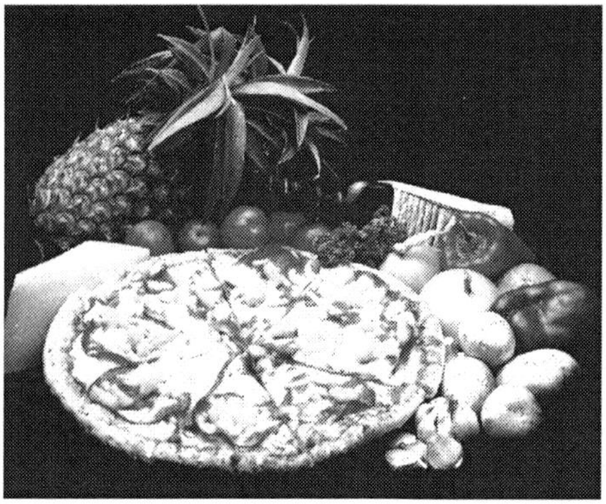

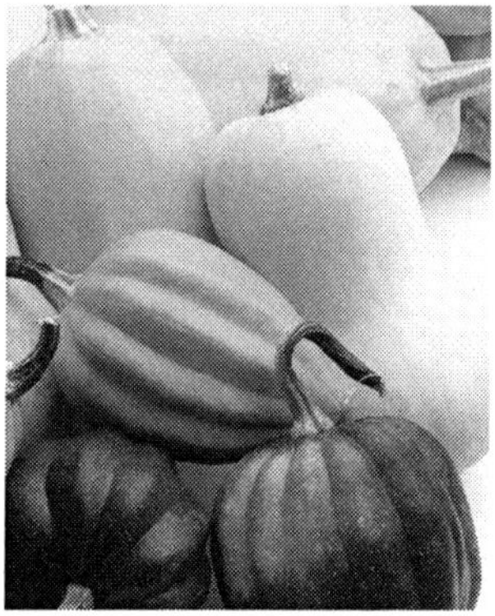

PUMPKIN BREAD	
Dry ingredients:	
2 tsp baking powder	1 tsp salt
½ cup maize meal (grits)	½ cup corn flour
2 cups oatmeal	3 tsp sesame seed (optional)
3 tsp linseed	
Mix dry ingredients together.	
Wet ingredients:	
2 eggs	3 Tbsp olive oil
½ cup milk or yogurt	1 heaped cup cooked mashed pumpkin
Mix wet ingredients together and add to dry ingredients. Bake in loaf (bread) pan at 180°C/350°F until cooked.	

POTATO FRITTERS	
3 medium sized potatoes	1 small grated onion
½ tsp raw brown sugar	2 eggs (beaten)
1 tsp baking powder	5 Tbsp corn flour
1 tsp salt	oil for frying
Grate potatoes and onions on fine side of grater. Add salt and sugar. Add eggs. Add flour and baking powder. Mix to a dropping consistency. Drop dessert spoonfuls into hot oil and fry until brown, turn over, fry and drain on absorbent paper.	

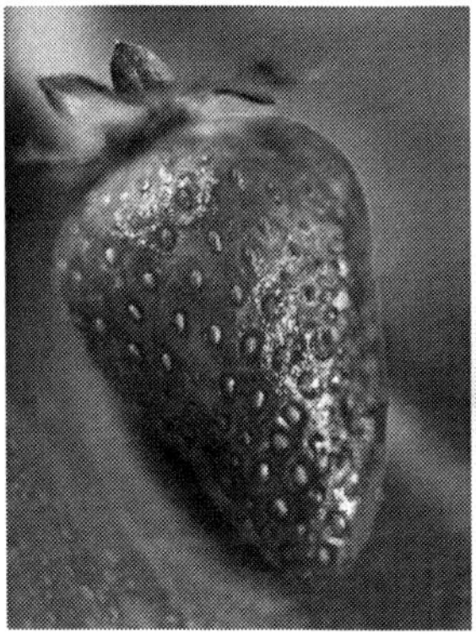
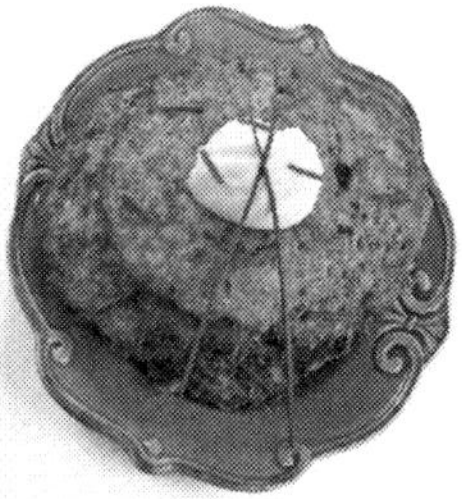
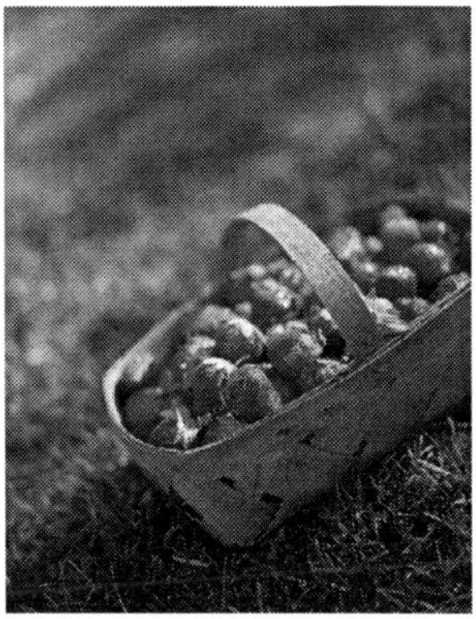

STRAWBERRY JAM	
1 cup fresh strawberries (or other preferred fruit)	
4 apples	1 tsp cinnamon
2 cups freshly squeezed orange juice	
Grate apples. Combine all ingredients in a saucepan. Gradually bring to the boil and simmer 30 minutes (or until thick). Store in airtight containers or jars and refrigerate.	

YOGURT (This is the only yogurt I recommend unless commercial yogurts are organic and contain live cultures. Avoid colored or flavored yogurt).
Boil 1 liter milk and leave to cool to body temperature (37ºC/98.6ºF).
Add 2 large tablespoons commercial unflavored yogurt made with live culture. Mix well.
Pour into either a flask (optional to pre-warm the flask by rinsing it with boiling water) or an ice bucket. Leave 6/8 hours or overnight. The flask method is more successful. Should you not have a flask or ice bucket, pour into a Pyrex dish, cover and place in warming drawer or very low oven (on warming temperature) for 6/8 hours or overnight. Refrigerate until set or eat immediately.
Eat unflavored or add either granola/muesli or oatmeal with fresh fruit, nuts, raw honey, etc., prior to serving.
Keep 2 tablespoons each time for starting off the next batch of yogurt. After a few batches (approx. 6) this will need replacing with 2 tablespoons commercial unflavored yogurt.
Important: Do not use thawed milk or get any water in the mixture.
Note: This recipe may also be used with commercial yogurt makers.

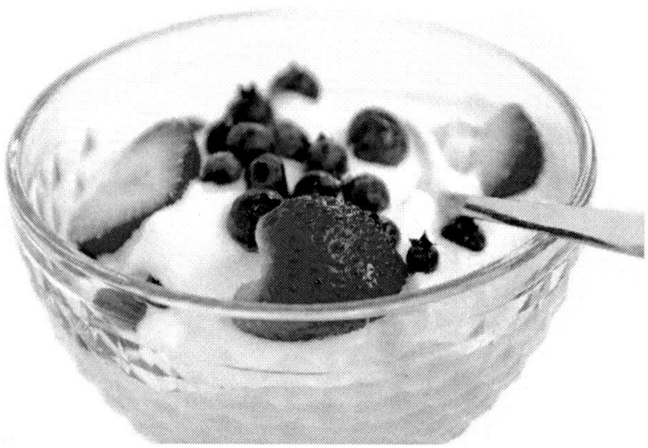

RAW FOOD RECIPES FOR BLENDER
No cooking required

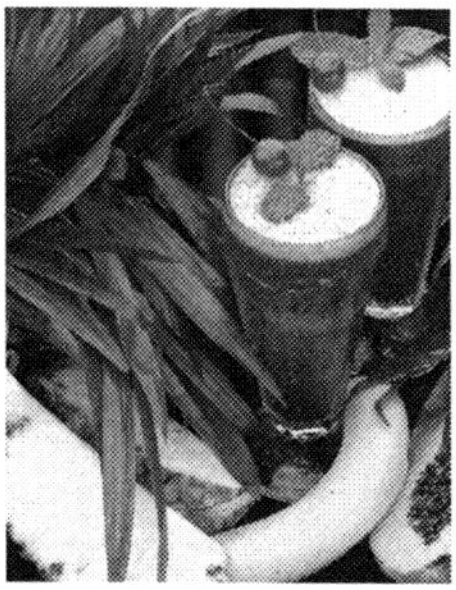

FRUIT DRINKS
1) Blend 2 bananas (or fruit of your preference) with 1 cup of plain, unflavored yogurt. Optional: add a little raw honey to sweeten.
2) Liquidize 2 bananas with 1 cup apple, grape, cranberry, peach, apricot, or other 100% commercial fruit juice.

FRUIT JUICES
1) Orange: Peel, cut and place in blender (with seeds); add ½ glass filtered water; pinch of All Spice - blend.
2) Apple, pear, pineapple, mango, kiwi, peach or any other fruit of your choice may be used as alternatives.
3) Mixed fruit cocktail: Combine any fruit of your choice and blend with ½ glass filtered water.
4) Watermelon: Blend without adding additional water.

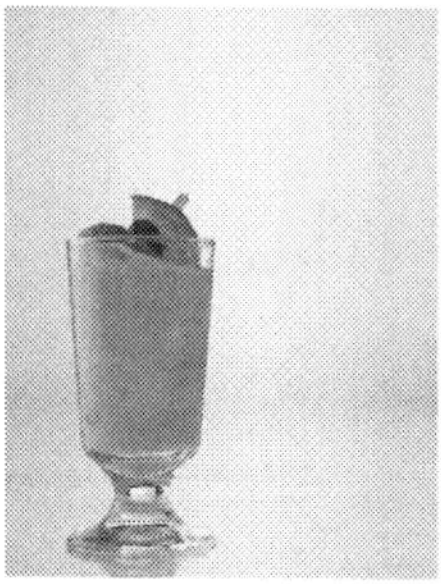

FRUIT SHAKE (FRUIT-LATA)
Blend a mixture of fruit (or use leftover fruit salad) with 1 cup of plain yoghurt and raw honey to taste. Optional: Add almonds

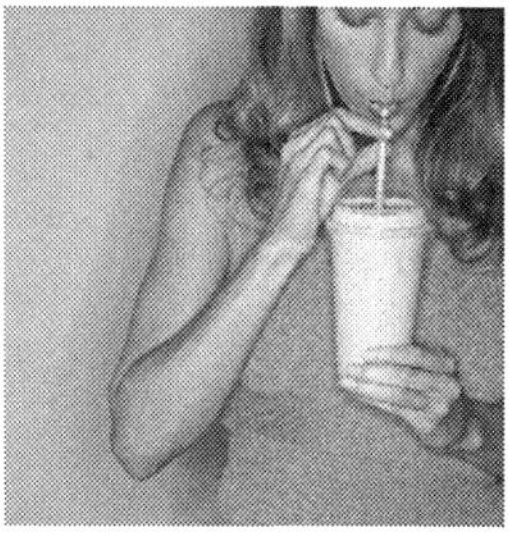

VANILLA ICE CREAM	
2 Banana	1 Tbsp raw honey (or to taste)
1 Cup plain yoghurt	1 cup ice
1 tsp Vanilla Extract (organic)	
Combine all ingredients in a blender and blend. Consistency should be that of ice cream otherwise add more ice.	

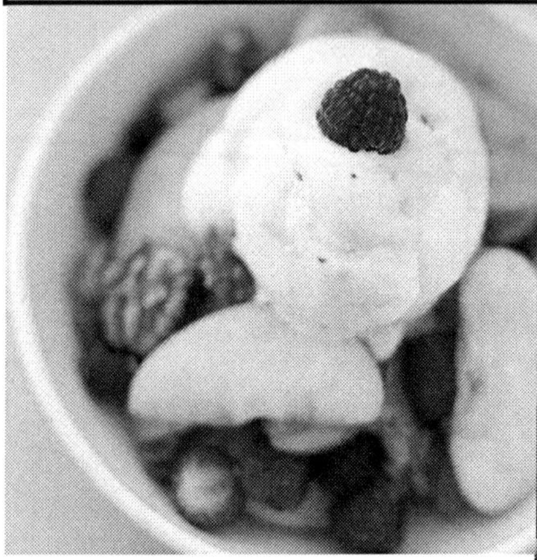

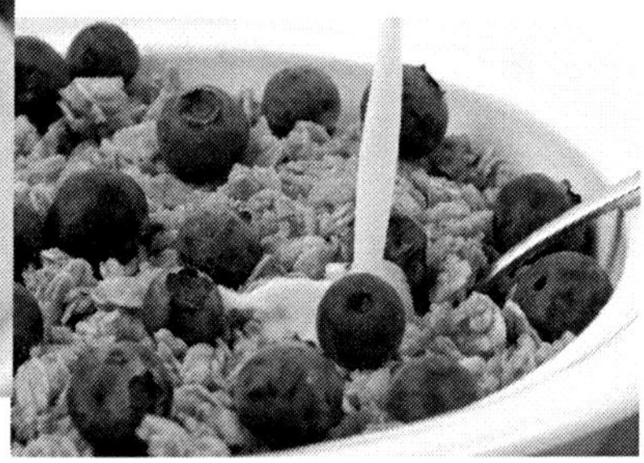

GRANOLA / MUESLI
Place a mixture of fruit in the blender (banana, apple, pear, pineapple, orange etc.). Wash and add 2 tablespoons each of sunflower seeds and raisins (or sultanas); Add nuts of your choice. Add ½ cup of oatmeal. Add plain yoghurt (or milk) and blend until required consistency obtained. Blend well for small children.

SOUP (WARM)
1) Raw Soup: Wash, peel and slice small portions of raw carrots, butternut, onions, cauliflower, broccoli, peas, and any other vegetable of your choice. 1 **cooked** potato - potato and sweet potatoes or yams are the only vegetables, which needs to be pre-cooked. Add 1 vegetable stock cube/bullion (or 1 tsp vegetable stock powder) and natural fresh herbs or vegetable salt seasoning. Peel and cut vegetables and place in blender with seasoning. Pour boiling water over and blend until smooth.
2) Cooked Soup: Store left-over cooked vegetables in air tight container and refrigerate. Use as soon as possible (do not keep for longer than 1 day). Make soup by placing left-over cooked vegetables in blender; add boiling water, season to taste and blend until desired consistency obtained. Warm slightly if necessary.

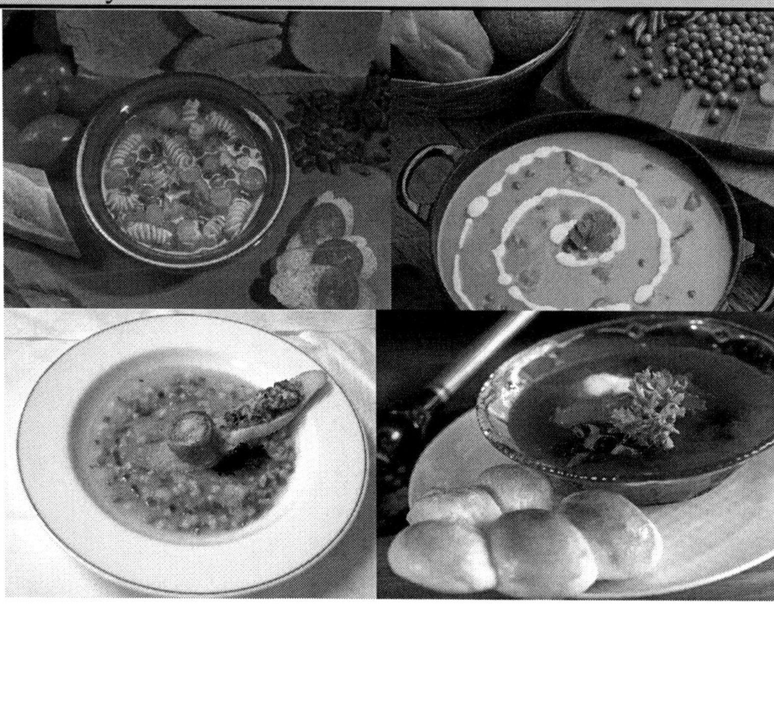

SOUP (COLD) OR DIP FOR VEGETABLE PLATTER
SOUP: Squeeze lemon juice over avocado to prevent it turning brown. Blend avocado and cucumber until correct consistency obtained for soup. Add seasoning.
DIP: To thicken for a dip, add smooth cottage cheese.
VEGETABLE PLATTER: Prepare carrot, cucumber, celery, raw butternut and radish sticks, wash baby tomatoes, flat peas in the pod, and break cauliflower and broccoli up into small sections.

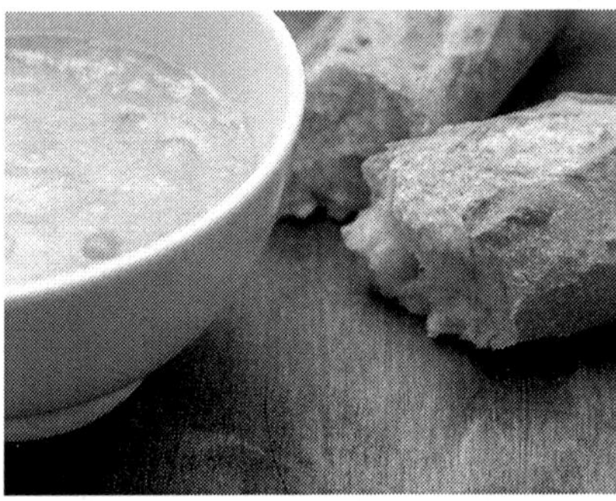
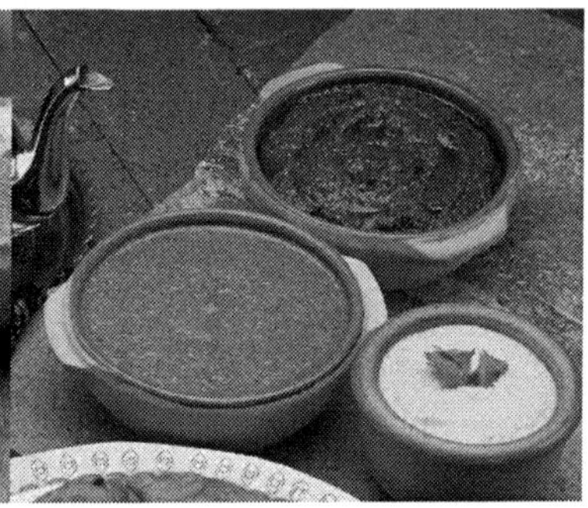

YOGURT
Blend: 1 cup milk with ½ lemon (juice and fiber) to sour.
Add fruit of your choice, to flavor. Serve as is or pour over granola/muesli or other fruit of your choice.

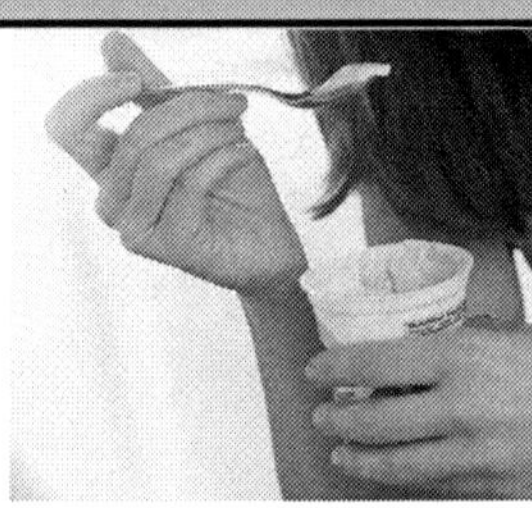

HEALTHY EATING - MADE EASY

The following recipes were submitted by Jessica Hart from *"Healthy Eating - Made Easy"*

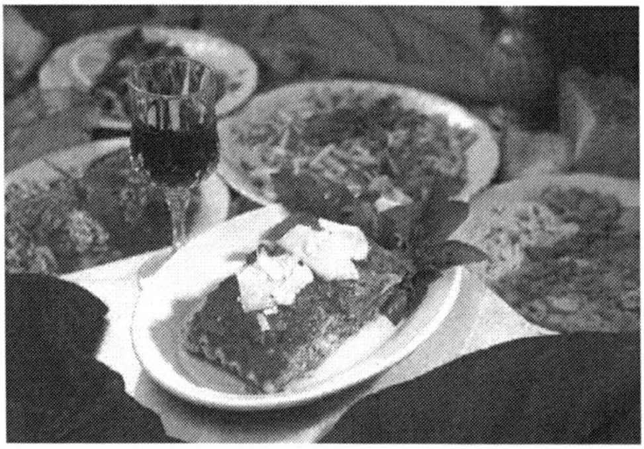

VEGETABLE LASAGNE (serves 8 - 10)	
60 ml cold pressed olive oil	3 medium onions sliced
2 ml curry powder	1 celery stalk sliced
500 ml grated butternut	3 cloves garlic (crushed)
10 ml mixed herbs	60 ml chopped fresh parsley
1,5 ml ground nutmeg	375 ml vegetable or chicken stock
400 g cooking tomatoes (peeled and chopped)	5 ml raw brown sugar
30 ml chopped fresh basil	30 ml corn flour

Sauté onion in olive oil; add curry powder and stir fry for 1 minute.
Add celery, butternut and garlic; stir fry for a further 2 minutes.
Add parsley and seasoning and stir until well mixed.
Add stock, tomatoes, basil and sugar.
Simmer slowly for 20 minutes.
Thicken with cornstarch.

White Sauce	
75 ml butter	75 ml corn flour
500 ml milk	salt, pepper
2.5 ml mustard powder	

Melt butter; add corn flour and cook gently for 1 minute, stirring. Add salt, pepper and mustard. Slowly add milk, stirring contiguously to prevent lumps forming; cook on low heat until thick.
400 g imported Italian Pasta (flat, shell or screw noodles). Cook according to instructions.
80 g grated mozzarella cheese
Spread a little white sauce on base of dish. Layer as follows: Pasta; vegetable mix; white sauce - repeat. Sprinkle grated cheese on top. Bake at 180°C/350°F for 30 minutes.

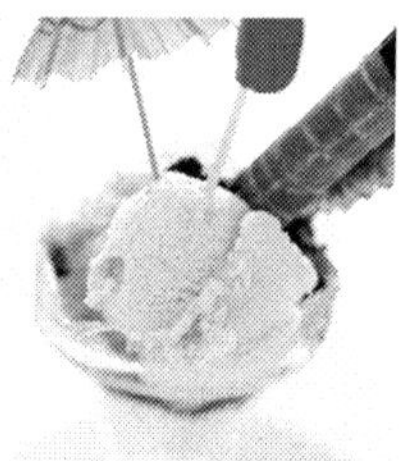

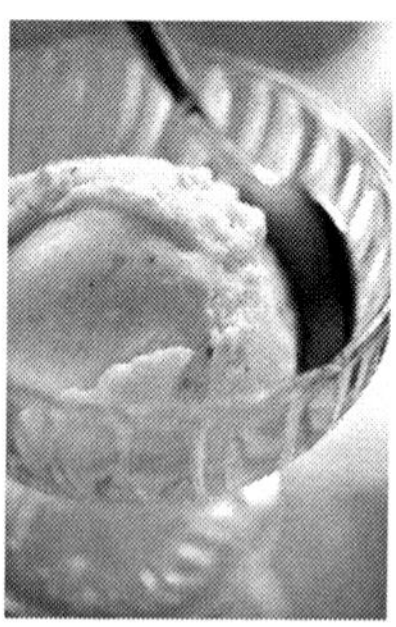

BANANA FROZEN YOGURT	
500 ml thick unflavored, plain yogurt	
180 ml raw honey	5 ml ground cinnamon
375 ml banana puree (made by mashing ripe bananas)	
1) Combine yogurt and honey and mix well. 2) Add cinnamon and banana. 3) Pour mixture into plastic container and freeze for 1 ½ hours. 4) Remove from freezer and beat until smooth. 5) Return to freezer for 1 hour then beat again. 6) Return to freezer and allow to set. 7) Serve with slices of fresh fruit.	

HEALTH BREAD	
2 cups brown rice flour	2 cups corn flour
1 x 500 ml carton unflavored yogurt	
8 ml salt	10 ml bicarbonate soda;
185 ml sunflower seeds	20 ml raw unfiltered honey
50 ml sesame and sunflower seeds for garnish	

1) Mix together flours, salt, honey and 185 ml sunflower seeds
2) Mix bicarbonate soda with a little yogurt, add to dry ingredients together with the remaining yogurt
3) Half fill yogurt container with water.
4) Slowly add water to remaining ingredients until flour is absorbed and dough is fairly wet.
5) Grease loaf (bread) pan and spoon dough into pan.
6) Sprinkle sesame and sunflower seeds over dough and drizzle a little warmed honey over the seeds.
7) Bake at 190ºC/375ºF for approximately 45 minutes to 1 hour.

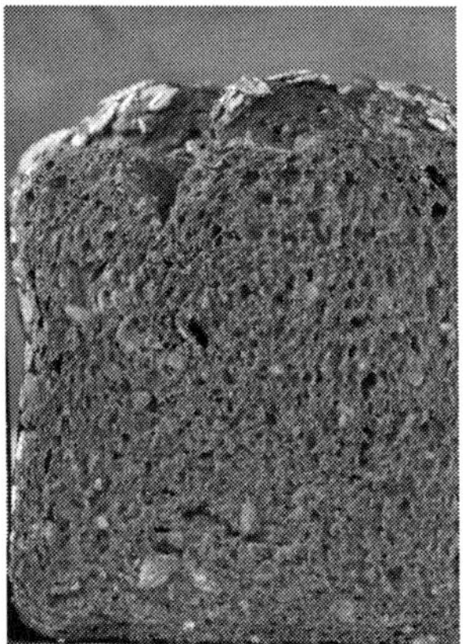

CHICKEN LIVER PATE	
1 tsp cold pressed olive oil	1 clove garlic (crushed)
1 large onion, finely chopped	5 ml mixed herbs
225 g chicken livers	15 ml brandy (optional)
1 ml paprika	
75 g smooth low-fat cottage cheese	
fresh parsley, chopped, and paprika to garnish	

1) Heat oil in thick-based pan and add 10 ml water. Add chopped onion, cover pan and cook gently for 3 minutes
2) Trim chicken livers of any green or black particles, add to onion and cook for a further 3 minutes.
3) Add garlic and herbs and cook for a further 3 minutes.
4) Place mixture in food processor and blend until smooth.
5) Stir in brandy, paprika and cottage cheese. Turn into small glass bowl and chill for about an hour.
6) Sprinkled pate´ with chopped parsley and paprika. Serve with rye bread, rye crackers, rice cakes and carrot, celery and cucumber sticks.

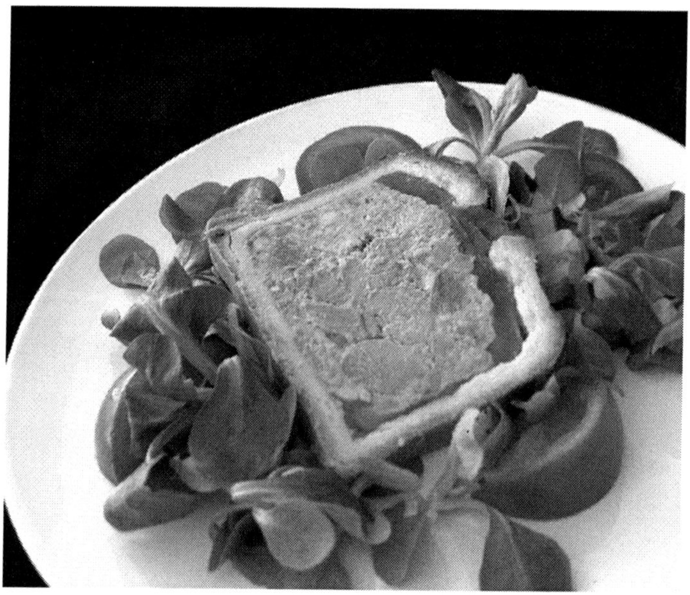

ONION SOUP (serves 4)	
30 ml cold pressed olive oil	750 ml chicken stock
3 large onions, peeled and sliced very thinly	30 ml corn flour
Grated cheese and chopped fresh parsley to garnish	

1) Heat oil in heavy based pan.
2) Toss onions in heated oil, and gently cook for approximately 10 minutes. Stir from time to time to ensure that the onions do not become too brown.
3) Add chicken stock and bring to boil, lower heat and allow to simmer for 10 minutes.
4) Mix a little cold water with the cornflour and pour into soup, stirring continuously to prevent lumps forming.
5) Simmer for a further 5 minutes.
6) Serve in soup bowls. Garnished with cheese and parsley

POTATO AND LEEK SOUP (serves 4)	
500 g potatoes, peeled and sliced	1 tsp finely chopped fresh mint
4 leeks, well washed and sliced into 2,5cm pieces	100 g chopped green onions
1 tsp finely chopped fresh dill	30 ml finely chopped fresh parsley

1) Boil potatoes and leeks for approximately 15 minutes in 4 cups water.
2) Allow to cool and transfer potatoes, leeks and cooking water plus dill and mint to blender and puree until smooth.
3) Pour back into pan and heat on low.
4) Add chopped green onions and cook for a further 10 minutes.
5) Serve sprinkled with chopped parsley.

SPINACH SALAD (RAW)	
4 large spinach leaves	100 g pecan nuts
1 large red apple	60 ml fresh lemon juice
2 stalks celery	200 ml unflavored yogurt
5 ml raw honey	

1) Wash spinach thoroughly in salt water, cut away from center stalk and spin leaves in a salad spinner.
2) Finely slice spinach.
3) Core apple and slice thinly - dip into lemon juice to prevent turning brown.
4) Slice celery stalks thinly.
5) Chop pecan nuts.
6) Combine lemon juice, yogurt and honey.
7) Layer spinach, apple, celery and pecan nuts in a glass bowl (repeat layers).
8) Prior to serving, pour yogurt mixture over salad as a dressing.

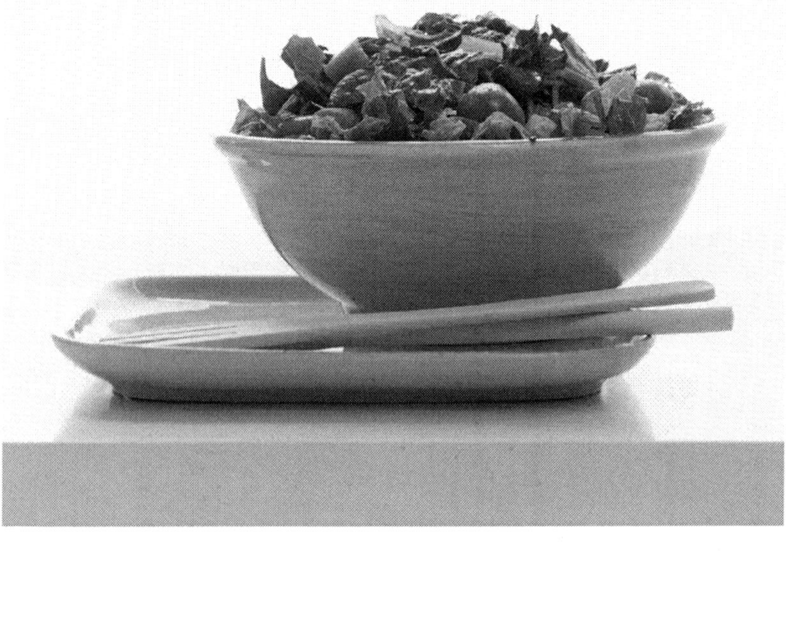

GRANOLA / MUESLI	
500 g raw oats (toasted in oven for 5 - 8 minutes at 100 ºC/200 ºF - shake periodically to prevent burning)	
250 ml sunflower seeds	250 ml linseeds
250 ml sesame seeds	
Blend seeds in a grinder or blender to break husks and release Gamma-linolenic acid (GLA)	
6 sun dried prunes chopped	6 sun dried apple rings chopped
4 - 6 sun dried peach halves chopped	4 - 6 sun dried pear halves chopped
250 ml mixed sun dried raisins, sultanas, currents	½ packet dates chopped
2 x 1 liter packets skim milk powder	

Mix all ingredients together and place in an airtight container.
Serve in breakfast bowl and pour boiling water over.
Allow to stand for 5 minutes to allow the oats to cook slightly.
Spoon 30 to 40 ml unflavored yogurt over serving and enjoy.
Optional extra: sliced fresh fruit can be added for additional fiber, vitamins and minerals.
Note: If granola/muesli is to be kept for more than 2 weeks store in the refrigerator as the GLA released from the seeds will turn rancid.

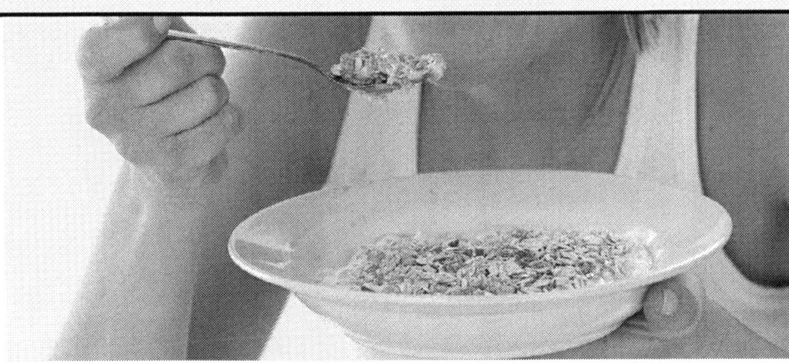

RECOMMENDED READING

(Some are "Golden Oldies" but the information is valuable!)

BOOKS ON *CANDIDA ALBICANS*

"Candida albicans - Could Yeast be Your Problem?" Leon Chaitow.
"Candida albicans, Yeast and Your Health" Gill Jacobs.
"Candida albicans, Yeast-free Recipes for Renewed Health and Vitality" Richard Turner and Elizabeth Sinonsen (excellent recipes).
"Candida Diet Against It" Dr. Luc De Schepper (excellent recipes).
"Coping with Candida" Shirley Trickett.
"The Candida albicans Yeast-free Cook Book" Pat Connolly.
"The Missing Diagnosis" Dr. Orian Truss.
"The Yeast Syndrome" John Parks Trowbridge.

BOOKS OF GENERAL INTEREST

"Aromatherapy for Natural Health and Beauty" Cecilia Salvesen.
"Ten Stages of Disease" Cecilia Salvesen
"Reflexology - A Practical Introduction" Inge Dougans
"Reflexology: Art, Science & History" Christine Issel
"Alkalize or Die" Dr. Theodore A. Baroody
"The Schwarzbein Principle" Diana Schwarzbein, M.D. & Nancy Deville
"The China Study" T. Colin Campbell, PhD cand Thomas M. Campbell II
"Green for Life" Vitoria Boutenko
"Fit for Life" Harvey and Marily Damond
"Diet, Crime and Delinquency" Alexander Schuss.
"Genetically Engineered Foods. Are they safe? You decide" Laura Ticciati and Robin Ticciati Ph.D.

INDEX

G

H

I

L

M

N

O

P

R

S

T

V

W

Z